I CHOOSE
TO LIVE

*A Journey
Through Life With ALS*

By William M. Sinton

I CHOOSE TO LIVE

A Journey
Through Life With ALS

First Printing/August 2002
Second Printing/August 2006

ISBN: 0-9706007-1-2
Library of Congress Catalog Card Number: 2002109638

Banbury Publishing, Inc.
36148 North Banbury Court
Gurnee, IL 60031

Printed in the U.S.A.

TABLE OF CONTENTS

Preface

First of all, I hope that I can be a motivation to those who are severely handicapped so that they can still enjoy life. I believe that I am still making useful contributions to the world. Not only have I written this book, but I am an active member of several radio clubs and have written articles for ham radio magazines and newsletters since acquiring ALS.

I believe I can give courage to caregivers of handicapped people. They can make a difference in helping others to live useful lives. I think that I can communicate a few of the things that my caregivers and I have learned about taking care of me. This has been and still is a learning process.

Also, I would like to tell people about the mysterious disease that is known as ALS, which stands for amyotrophic lateral sclerosis, but which is most often known as Lou Gehrig's disease in the U.S.

I have been inspired by numerous books I've read since acquiring ALS. The book that made the biggest impression on me was "Tuesdays with Morrie" by Mitch Albom. My wife, Marge, read it to me and we were often brought to tears by this sad story. Stephen Hawking has also been provocative. I have listened to his book "A Brief History of Time" on audiotape. In fact, I listened to it twice. I also listened to his other book "Black Holes and Baby Universes and Other Essays." He also has a movie called "A Brief History of Time." Other books that I found stimulating are "Journeys with ALS," which contains brief histories of persons with ALS, and "In Sunshine and Shadow," which is a collection of short stories about people with ALS published by the Keith Worthington ALS Society. The foreword by Stephen Hawking was particularly encouraging. Another book is "Charlie's Victory" by Charlie and Lucy Wedemeyer. This is a story of the amazing courage and determination by a victim of this awful disease.

I have also been reassured by other books written by people who have suffered from severe paralyzing diseases and injuries. An important book is "Still Me" by Christopher Reeve. He tells a lot about how he and his wife have dealt with his injuries and how he has learned to cope with being on a ventilator. Reeve's remake of the movie "Rear Window" is interesting for its portrayal of the needs of someone who is on a ventilator. The ventilator shown in the movie is exactly like the one I am on. Another book, which was the direct motivation for writing this book, is "The Diving Bell and the Butterfly" by Jean Dominique Bauby. This is the story about a man who suffered a severe stroke while in the prime of his life. A book about a teenager who coped with a broken neck is "Rescuing Jeffrey" by his father, Richard Galli.

I am indebted to many people who have helped me. The people who have given me the most personal attention are my caregivers, Tina Winscott, Lee Mitchelson, Tina Haver, and Barbara Redsteer. They take care of my every need during the days of the week. Marge helps me at night and on weekends. Sometimes Marge is off on vacation and my caregivers are with me all the time. I owe much to these caring people. I am very grateful to the Patient Services Coordinators of the Valley of the Sun ALS Association. Specifically they are Don Long, the late Mary Lois Long, Carol Antly, Dawn Butler, Marilyn Laird, and Jo Tanzer who have driven to Flagstaff from Phoenix to facilitate an ALS support group meeting.

One of the things that has made writing this book possible is the IBM program called "ViaVoice." It was advertised on TV with the slogan "I talk, it types." It really works. I have only to talk into a microphone and it types what I say. It sometimes comes out with amusing mistakes. I once said "I went up Mount Wilson with John Strong," which it interpreted as "I went up Mount Wilson with guns drawn." The only problem I have experienced with it has been in making corrections. It often screws it up worse than it was. The program runs on my "Special Edition" iMac computer. I have used Headmaster Plus made by Prentke Romich to make editing corrections. This device sits on my head like headphones and moves the cursor through an infrared beam as I move my head.

I am indebted to the following persons who have contributed to this book: Lydia Broussard, June King, Len Koel, Lee Mitchelson, Barbara Redsteer, Jane Spencer, John Spencer and Tina Winscott.

I am especially indebted to Lissy Peace of Blanco and Peace Enterprises for seeing this book through to publication.

William M. Sinton
April, 2001

Medical Personnel I Liked

Kim Allen, Speech Therapist
Joseph Colorafi, MD - Pulmonologist
Stephanie Effinger, Respiratory Therapist
Kenneth Epstein, MD - Specialist
Michael Flores, MD - Primary Care

Melissa Hough, PT - Physical Therapist
Jerry Mohr, MD - Surgeon
Stephen Ritland, MD - Neurosurgeon
Lawrence Stern, MD - Neurologist
Michael Vengrow, MD - Neurologist

My Personal Caregivers

Tina Haver
Lee Mitchelson, CNA, CC/RSA
Barbara Redsteer
Tina Winscott

This Book is Dedicated to Marge

Throughout our more than forty years of marriage, our love has grown stronger and stronger. ALS has put severe strains on this bond. Being my primary caregiver these last seven years has been a huge burden on her. But our mutual love has reverberated between us, sometimes strained, but always renewed.

Marge, I love you with all my heart, body, and soul.

Bill

Beginning To Stumble

In October 1992, while on one of our evening walks, I mentioned to Marge that I was walking funny. I didn't think too much about it at the time and I didn't worry either because it seemed like such a simple thing. But by Christmas, I was getting a little worse. Still, with my aging (I was now 67), I didn't worry much about it.

My sons were home for Christmas and I didn't have much time to think about my problems. My eldest son, Bob, urged me to get my amateur radio license renewed. I let it lapse more than forty years earlier. He got his ham license about two years previously so I took his suggestion seriously and began studying for mine. There were two general tasks I had to do. One was to master Morse code and the other was to learn all of the written parts of the exam that I would have to take. In two or three weeks, I was ready to take exams. I took and passed all of the exams except the written one that would have qualified me for the extra class license, which is the highest ham license that one can get. I didn't take this last exam because I had not studied for it at all. About six months later I took and passed the final exam.

I was a frequent blood donor and over the years I have donated close to four gallons. In February, I went to donate blood and they found that my blood pressure was too high for me to donate further. I immediately made an appointment to see my primary care doctor. In his office, my blood pressure was down to its normal count. Apparently, they call this condition labile high blood pressure when the blood pressure is not continuously high. It is not of too much concern so he and I didn't worry about it. I mentioned to him about my troubles with walking and by this time, I was also having trouble getting up from a chair. In retrospect, his response to this was most surprising. He immediately jumped to the conclusion that I had spinal stenosis, a narrowing of the channel through the backbone for the spinal cord. At the time I had never heard of this. He ordered an X-ray and sent me off to radiology.

I came back a few days later to review the X-rays with him. The conclusion of the radiologists was that the X-rays were consistent with a diagnosis of spinal stenosis. This, of course, was the suspected diagnosis he had listed on the X-ray order. He also sent me to see Dr. Mark Donnelly, a vascular surgeon, to test whether the circulation in my legs was adequate. That, it turned out, wasn't the problem.

At this point, Marge and I had a tremendous vacation planned. We drove down to Phoenix and the next day we took an Amtrak train to New Orleans. After spending the night in a hotel in the French Quarter, we embarked the next day on the Delta Queen for a 7-day trip up the Mississippi River with stops at various locations on the way for day tours. We turned around at Vicksburg and headed back to New Orleans. I enjoyed being on this boat because it was a steamboat, and steam engines were one of my hobbies. Even before it left the dock, I went down to the engine room and told the enginemen of my interest in live steam. They showed me the engines and then led me off to the boiler room. I had a grand tour of the innards of the boat.

While in New Orleans, one day I stumbled at a slight unevenness of the pavement and fell headlong on my face. Fortunately, I didn't bang myself up badly. I also fell again at one of the day tours. One of the fellow passengers picked me up. One thing that I began to notice nearly every time I fell is that a "helpful person" will immediately start to pull you to your feet without checking whether you might have injuries or not. It is most disconcerting when you don't know whether or not you've been hurt. I noticed that my legs were getting weaker because coming up the stairs from the dining room I had to pull myself up each step with the railing. I also remember falling another time when I didn't pick my foot up enough to get it over the 4-inch high lip at the doorway to our stateroom. Fortunately, on this fall there was a bed in front of me and I fell flat on that.

When I returned to Flagstaff, my doctor sent me off to get a CT scan of the lumbar region of my spine. Again, the results were consistent with the diagnosis of spinal stenosis. He was now sure that that is what I had. It scared me. He sent me to Dr. Steve Ritland, a neurosurgeon who sent me to get an MRI of my neck. I was now getting very concerned. However, my philosophy has always been that things will come out all right in the end so don't worry about it.

The next thing that happened after I was back in Flagstaff was a stroke of luck. I developed a case of hives all over my body and so I made an appointment to see Dr. Kenneth Epstein, an immunologist. He happened to work in the same office as my primary care physician and so he had access to my medical records. The appointment wasn't for three of four days and by that time all my hives were gone. I went to see him anyway and, as it turned out, he wanted to see me because of the medical records about my back. He apparently realized it wasn't my back and sent me to get an EMG. An EMG is an electro-myogram which is a combination of measuring electrical impulses in the nerves by inserting tiny needles into the arms or legs and also measuring the reaction of the muscles to electrical shocks. The impulses from the nerves were recorded by computer but they also came out of a loudspeaker so that the doctor and I could hear them.

Dr. Leddington, who practices physical medicine, began measuring the responses in my legs. When he measured nerve responses with a needle stuck in various places, he would ask me to tighten the appropriate muscle. I would hear steady buzzes as I tightened the muscle. When my muscle was relaxed I would hear a popping sound.

He spent some time giving me electrical shocks, which I loathed. I had an aversion to them from working on radios. I remember getting shocked twice in a row from 800 volts. Most people don't like the needles, but I don't like the shocks. Everyone finds that the EMGs are very unpleasant.

When he started on my arms and put the needles in to measure the electrical activity of my nerves, he told me to relax my arm as much as possible. But I could still hear the pop, pop, pop of the electrical impulses in my nerves. He again told me to relax but still the pop, pop, pop went on, maybe somewhat slower, but still pop, pop, pop. He said, "Oh, I didn't expect that."

At my next visit with Dr. Ritland, he looked at the MRI and the CT scan and then asked me to walk across the floor. Then he said that he didn't see enough in any of my vertebrae to cause my problems. That definitely ruled out spinal stenosis. But by this time, Marge had started a file folder that she called "Bill's Back." Subsequently, everything that related to my condition went into this folder about "Bill's Back."

Dr. Epstein and I went over the results of the EMG. He was confused by the chart sent by the doctor who did the exam and it surely was confusing to me. He then thought that I should get a muscle biopsy. For this procedure I had to go down to a clinic in Phoenix that specializes in muscle and nerve medicine. It was an outpatient procedure to extract a half-inch by half-inch by one-inch segment of the muscle in my thigh. They gave me a local anesthetic and a shot that would make me sleepy. I guess I fell asleep and didn't wake up for probably about an hour. When I did, Marge was at my side and I was free to go. I hobbled out of the clinic and we went out to eat. The next day we drove back to Flagstaff. It would take some time to get the results from the examination of the thigh muscle biopsy. The muscle segment would have to be frozen and sliced with a microtome and then stained and examined under a microscope.

Meanwhile, I had received my ham license in the mail. After a few weeks, I acquired a handy-talky for the amateur radio bands and got busy using that.

The amateur radio Field Day was on the last weekend in June. This is a contest where amateur radio clubs all over the U.S. and Canada go out into the field to try out their equipment under simulated emergency conditions. All equipment is powered by batteries, gasoline generators, solar cells, wind generators, and sometimes even water power. I had become a member of the Coconino Amateur Radio Club. They went out into the U.S. Forest at a spot about eight miles north of Flagstaff.

The spot was very rutty from trucks having driven there when the ground was very soggy in the springtime. I was stumbling badly on the tire tracks. Marge left me there while she went back to our house to get me a cane. Meanwhile, I helped others set up their equipment.

That night we camped in a tent in the forest. I remembered that it got very cold even in June, but that's Flagstaff. We got out the space blankets and finally got warm. I remember that our cots were very noisy when you rolled over. Despite my stumbling, I had a great time. I spent my time at the Morse code station and although I didn't operate the radio, I did keep a log of the radio contacts that were made during the day.

Dr. Epstein suggested that I make an appointment with Dr. Vengrow, a neurologist in Flagstaff. When I arrived at the appointed time, Dr. Vengrow had all of the results of the previous tests available. He reviewed them and then got out his little hammer and, after I had crossed my legs, he hit me on the knee. He then asked me to take off my shoes and socks. With an object from his pocket, which he said was the key to his Mercedes Benz, he rubbed - no, forcibly scribed - the bottom of my foot. This test, which excites the plantar nerve, is known as the Babinski reflex. I later learned that the movement of the big toe, whether up or down or not at all or how much, can tell a lot about the central nervous system. He told me to put my shoe and sock back on and meanwhile, he went across the hall to his office. I think that all doctors should know this test as well as the hammer on the the knee test. It would have told my primary care physician that it was not spinal stenosis that I had.

Dr. Vengrow called me over to his office in a few minutes. He said that I had a motor neuron disease and mumbled something about not having bulbar involvement. I noticed that he had a textbook open to a chapter on ALS. He asked me to schedule another appointment so that he could do his own EMG testing because the previous test left some unanswered questions. So I came back again, and after putting me through more shocks and needle sticks, he then said that he would like me to see a neurologist at the University Medical Center in Tucson. The name of this neurologist was Dr. Lawrence Stern. He would be my neurologist for at least the next five years.

All of this left me very scared, but I remained optimistic. I had always thought that the things that I worry about are not in my future.

I Choose To Live

Life is Where You Find It

"I've learned:
That to ignore the facts does not change
the facts".

Andy Rooney

I have ALS.   I put this up front to acknowledge that I am no longer suffering from denial. I don't believe that my denial period was very long.   I want to stress that getting over denial quickly is important with any disease. Doing this has enabled me to cope with my disabilities.

ALS is generally known as Lou Gehrig's disease in the U.S., motor neurone disease in the U.K., and maladie de Charcot in French-speaking countries. ALS stands for amyotrophic lateral sclerosis. Amyotrophic means no muscle nourishment, hence, muscle wasting. Lateral refers to the sides of the spinal column where the motor nerves are, and sclerosis means scarring or hardening. The British term, motor neurone disease, is much more descriptive to lay persons.   Persons with ALS are often referred to as PALS.

ALS is a terrible disease that generally doesn't strike until people are over 40. The disease progresses rapidly and is almost always fatal in a period of two to five years. It attacks the nerves that conduct the impulses from the brain to the muscles. These nerves die and do not regenerate. Generally, it begins when weakness develops in the hands and moves up the arms and then involves feet and legs. Soon, muscles in the neck, tongue, and those in the chest and abdomen that are required for respiration, become affected. Sometimes the feet and legs are weakened first. In other cases, the tongue and swallowing muscles are involved first. This last case is called bulbar onset and with it the progression is most rapid and death usually follows in one to three years. The rate of progression varies widely from one case to another. The expressed symptoms of the disease also vary widely between cases. Many with bulbar onset will show incessant drooling. But I've never experienced this.

ALS not only afflicts the person whom it strikes, but all the family members, the spouse, the parents, the children, and the brothers and sisters. All these people are emotionally involved from seeing their loved one waste away and they are often called upon to provide the caregiving that the PALS require. It places tremendous stress on family ties.

About 5% to 10% of ALS cases are of genetic origin. These are called FALS for familial ALS, while the others are called sporadic ALS, or SALS, for short. Recently, a gene defect has been found to be responsible for at least some of the FALS cases. But the cause of the remainder of the cases is unknown, and there is no cure or effective treatment for either kind of ALS. There are about 5000 new cases of ALS each year and at any time there are about 25,000 cases in the U.S. The disease is more frequent in men than women.

Many causes of SALS have been proposed, but none of these has been proved to be applicable. Actually, there are many possible causes, and I believe that ALS is not one disease but maybe several. The pathways, however, are undoubtedly similar. I find that I had been

10

exposed to many of the suggested pathogens. A number of a causative agents have been proposed to explain sporadic ALS. These include:

1. A slow-acting virus.
2. Poisoning from heavy metals.
3. Solvents, pesticides, and environmental poisons.
4. Previous trauma such as from severe injury.
5. Apoptosis, which means programmed cell death.
6. A bacterial infection.

There is a phenomenon, called post-polio syndrome, that mimics the paralytic effects of ALS. And there is also the possibility of other slowly acting viruses. There has been some recent work on this possibility. This new work will be discussed further in the next to last chapter.

A lot of discussion has been made lately about mercury amalgams in an e-mail newsletter devoted to ALS (see Bob Broedel in Appendix C). The American Dental Association says that the mercury level in the body from dental amalgams is far below toxic levels. Some say that just a little bit of mercury might cause effects that are below the levels considered as toxic. Others say that the dose makes the poison. That is, levels that are far below the level that is toxic are ineffective in causing SALS. The form of the mercury is of importance here. Mercury in organic compounds is far more toxic than are inorganic compounds of mercury, which are more toxic than mercury metal.

I believe that I have had contact with a number of the enumerated causes listed above. I certainly have had a large cumulative dose of heavy metals. Perhaps I was exposed to the polio virus. I have encountered a number of solvents since I've used benzene, acetone, methyl ethyl ketone, carbon tetrachloride, petroleum ethers, and many others. I also have had a severe injury to my leg that injured a nerve as the sensation in one area of my foot was deadened.

One area of research has been looking at clusters of ALS cases. A cluster is where a number of cases occur in the same locality or industry. Then, perhaps, a common factor can be found. One such occurrence was with the 49ers football team and their groundskeepers. There were three cases. It could be supposed that something like pesticide or herbicides put on the grass of the field was a common factor. However, three cases in 100 turns out not to be statistically significant since there are many groups of 100 in the U.S. each of which could have three cases. A number of veterans from the Gulf War have developed ALS. It is not yet determined whether this number is greater than the expected occurrences of ALS. However, it does seem that this is an important avenue for research.

Most of this book is autobiographical as I bring out many of these exposures to chemicals and past diseases. Some people, and I guess I may be one, have lived for a rather long time with the disease. Stephen Hawking, a famous cosmologist, and the late Senator Jacob Javits are two of these people. I have had this disease for eight years. I consider myself lucky because many, in fact most people who get ALS have only a few years to look forward to. When I was first diagnosed I thought I might have four years to live. I looked at this as being a good sign. I could count on four years! This gave me time to put my affairs in order.

I hope that in this book I will encourage those who have a debilitating disease that they have a good life to look forward to. In retrospect my past seven years have been full of life. I have enjoyed my hobbies, I have served, and still serve, on the Advisory Board of Lowell Observatory, I have been president of a ham radio club and my wife and I have traveled a fair amount and have enjoyed this much.

As I began to lose my abilities I realized that I should not dwell on what I had lost, but rather, I tried to look at what I could do. There are many things that we, as humans cannot do. We cannot swim like a fish, we cannot fly like a bird, and we cannot burrow through the ground like a mole. We don't worry about not doing those things. With that in mind, I don't worry about those things that I no longer can do, but I look for those things that I can do. With the aid of computers I can do many things. I wrote this book without lifting a finger, a thing that I can't do. I get out and travel some and have even made cross-country trips. My wife and I go out to eat about once a week. I go downtown and have coffee with my cronies about once a week.

I know that many people, when faced with a situation such as mine, have chosen to end their lives. I think that is their choice. Many with ALS have chosen to make this choice. A PALS was shown on national TV taking his life with help from Dr. Kevorkian. I certainly have thought about doing this. I have considered suicide twice in my life, while in college and again when I began losing mobility about five years ago. But dying like this is an offense against those who are living. With a lot of help from friends, caregivers, and my wife and with my own courage, I do not choose to do this. There are so many things that are interesting in life that I look forward to each day.

I hope too, that this book will be beneficial to those who are in need of some ideas on how to cope with disabilities. It has been a great learning experience for me and my wife. There are no single solutions that fit all. We have only learned by trial and error and many times had to go back and rethink things. Maybe some of the ideas that I have included here will be a start.

Some of My Earliest Memories

The choo-choo train ran all are around the track.
oo-oo Ooo-oo Oooo-oo.
(part of lullaby)

My mother told me that I was born in the front bedroom of our brick hipped-roof bungalow. My birth was attended by Dr. Wantz. He was a family physician who lived about ten blocks away. I remember that when I was sick he would always come with his little black bag that contained his stethoscope and other paraphernalia and with another black case that contained many vials of pills.

The brick house was built by my grandfather. He and my grandmother and an uncle, his wife, and their son lived in a house that was about six blocks away from us. At the time that these houses were built, the neighborhood was outside of the City of Baltimore, but Baltimore city limits were later extended and included this neighborhood. The region was called Mount Washington and was then the village of Mount Washington, but now is just an area of the city.

My mother told me that when I was several years old I caught diphtheria. Fortunately, Dr. Wantz had the serum that he had saved from his military service. My mother always told me that I caught diphtheria from eating snow. Today, this seems very unlikely to me. Anyhow, I am glad that I recovered from diphtheria.

I can remember my mother singing me a lullaby about a train running around a track. I can't remember all

15

the words now, but some of them are at the beginning of this chapter. I do remember that my mother told me that she would think I was asleep and would stop singing, but I would always say, "More mommy, more mommy."

I can remember that sometimes when my father came home from work, he would take me down to the railroad station in the village to see the commuter trains come through so I could wave to the engineers. The tracks that came through the village were part of the Pennsylvania Railroad and went on up to Harrisburg, Pennsylvania.

It seems that whenever Christmas came around I was always sick with the croup, or the grippe. I remember that at one of my early Christmases I received a windup train that ran on tracks I could hook together. Oh, was I thrilled at that! We had an electric train set that ran around a Christmas tree, but the windup was my train.

I can just barely remember a trip that we took to Hershey, Pennsylvania. I remember seeing a tremendous sunset on the way. But one thing that impressed me was an amusement park. One of the rides there was a miniature steam train. I had never seen one before. Of course, I clamored to ride it. I remember my father putting me up in one of the cars. I don't remember that ride too well. But I do remember the steam.

I can remember puzzling over what happened to mail that was put into a mailbox. In those days, the walk to a mailbox was rarely more than two or three blocks. A mailbox was about 18 inches high, 14 inches wide, and about 6 inches deep. The mailbox was mounted on a post that went down into the ground. I never saw anybody take mail out of the box, so I developed a theory that the mail went down the post, which I presumed was a pipe, down into the ground to another pipe like a sewer line. I imagined that a letter floated on water to the post office.

I remember being confused by radio. I could not imagine how the voices and music got into the radio set (that's what they were called in those days). I remember a radio set that my father built. It had just two tubes. The radio had a bakelite front panel, which was mounted at right angles to a piece of board that was actually a breadboard. The components that had knobs and dials were mounted on the bakelite panel, and components such as a tube socket were screwed to the breadboard. The wires that connected these components consisted of bus bars about 1/16-inch diameter. They were laid out very neatly with right-angle bends. Where they crossed, a short length of insulating tubing covered one of the wires. I later learned that this was called spaghetti tubing. It was all very neat and esthetically pleasing. It was actually very artful.

Batteries were used to power the radio. There were two kinds of batteries, the A batteries powered the filaments of the tubes, and the B battery, which was either 45 or 90 volts, supplied the main power for the radio. I remember seeing a Neutrodyne radio down in my basement. This radio was about two feet long and had about five large dials on the front, which all had to be tuned independently.

My great aunt, Amy, had a shore place where she also had a battery-powered radio. A car battery was used to power the filaments. The car battery was very messy with acid deposits on its top and sides. I was told to stay away from it. My great uncle, Cuno Rudolph, was a vice president of the Second National Bank of Washington D.C. and he was also one of the commissioners of Washington. At that time Washington didn't have a mayor, but rather had three commissioners appointed by the U.S. Congress. I remember a feeling of loss when my uncle Cuno died suddenly from a heart attack. I remember that my mother instructed my brother and me to pronounce Aunt Amy as "awnt" Amy and not "ant" Amy. I think that the fact that they had money had something to do with this.

In 1933, a major hurricane struck the Mid-Atlantic States. Trees were knocked down all around my neighborhood. My aunt's place on the Chesapeake Bay had been flooded. She had tried to escape in her chauffeured Lincoln, which had become mired in the flood and she had to hike to a nearby farmhouse. My parents, because we sometimes went down to her shore place on weekends, were expected to help clean and fix up after the storm damage. When we arrived, there was no electric power. I went out to the garage with my aunt's chauffeur. He was going to start up the emergency generator. I imagine now, that an emergency generator was an unusual thing to have at that time. Anyhow, I was very impressed with the generator and the storage batteries to be charged.

At some time I got a crystal set. The crystal set required a rather long length of wire for the antenna which my father put up. The crystal set had a large coil of tightly wound enameled wire. The insulation had been scraped off along one side of the coil and a slider contact was used to tune the radio. The tuning was not very selective and only about two stations could be tuned in. The crystal was a piece of galena that was mounted in a cylindrical piece of lead. There was a short wire, called a cat's whisker, that made contact with the bare part of the galena. It was very tricky to find a spot with the cat's whisker on the galena that would make the radio work. The crystal set had no batteries but required earphones. Imagine, all of the sound energy coming from the earphones was produced initially by the radio station.

Later on my friend Lee, who lived next door, and I set up a telephone line between our two houses. I believe I used my earphone as both the listening phone and the talking phone. I'm not sure what he used, but I think that at that point we didn't have real telephone equipment. We called ourselves the Bill-Lee Telephone Company.

I find it curious that hobbies and interests like radio and railroads have stayed with me throughout my life. At least in my case, early environments had a lot to do with my future interests.

I Choose To Live

Circa Age 11

"I've learned:
That simple walks with my father around the block
on summer nights when I was a child, did wonders
for me as an adult."

Andy Rooney

"Oops," I said as I dropped the precious droplet of mercury on the floor. I had reclaimed this from a broken thermometer that my father had saved for me. Now there were myriads of sparkling points of light on the floorboards. I went off to find a piece of typewriter paper. Returning with the paper, I scraped the tiny spheres of mercury together with the edge of the paper. The ball of mercury got bigger and it got easier to gather up more of the tiny spheres making an even bigger ball. Now I could push the ball along the crack in the floorboards and could pick up even more droplets until I recovered most of the original amount of mercury.

But while my original droplet of mercury was clean and shiny, this recovered droplet was all dirty and gray. But I knew what to do. I took out my handkerchief and put the ball of mercury in the middle of it and then I squeezed it through the handkerchief onto the piece of paper. The mercury was now clean but there was a dark spot in the middle of my handkerchief. I stuffed my handkerchief back into my pocket. I took out a dime. I put the droplet of mercury on the dime and rubbed it around vigorously and the dime became all shiny and bright. "Oh boy!" I put the dime back into my pocket.

21

The next day I was walking to school, a distance of about a half a mile. My older brother had told me about finding the square root of numbers. It looked something like long division, but one did funny things to the number in front of the long division sign. I couldn't remember the details. But I knew that the square root of 2 is 1.414. It occurred to me that 1 was too small to be the square root of 2 and that 2 was too large to be the square root of 2. If I were to average the two numbers, the result, 1 ½ , was closer to the square root of 2. Now if I divided 1 ½ into 2, the result would be 4/3. If I averaged 1 ½ and 4/3, the result, 17/12, which is the same as 1.4166 . . . is very much closer to the square root of 2. Wow! I believed I was on the right track. I supposed that if I were to keep on dividing my new answer into 2 and averaging the result with the previous answer, I would get closer and closer to the square root of 2. Many years later, I learned that a Hebrew mathematician did this about 2000 years B.C.

Later, I took the dime out of my pocket and it was all dirty and gray. I took out my handkerchief and rubbed the dime and it became bright again and the handkerchief became dirtier. About this time, I arrived at school and I put the dime and the handkerchief in my pocket.

I was fascinated with some of the things that animals could do that I couldn't do. One of these was flying like a bird. This was a time when airplanes were relatively new. My older brother Bob, who was about six years older than me, was very excited about flying and some of his interest rubbed off on me. We lived near to a small airport and airplanes frequently flew over our house. Bob and I would run outside to see them. Sometimes on Sundays, Dad would drive us to the airport so we could watch them take off and land. Sometimes we were allowed to walk right up to them. All of these planes were made of fabric that was stretched over a wooden framework. This type of construction was used for flying model aircraft (and still is). Not surprisingly, I tried to build a plane I could fly in! I only got a few sticks nailed together before my father put a stop to the project.

Another of my dreams was to burrow underground like a mole (we had moles in the backyard). I wanted to be able to burrow and come up in the fenced backyard of a friend. I eventually gave up these dreams of flying and burrowing. I came back to these reluctantly given up fantasies when I began to lose, one by one, my human abilities to ALS.

At another time, Bob let me go along with him when he went to his friend's house. His friend, Harwood, was an amateur radio operator. We went into his ham shack, that is what the radio amateurs call the place where they have their equipment. I was awed. Besides the strange looking radio equipment that I had not seen before, there were postcard-sized cards on the wall that confirmed radio contacts that Harwood had made with other hams all over the world. I can still remember one from Ireland. I didn't know that one could have a hobby like this. Seeing the ham radio gear rekindled my interest in my crystal set. When I got home, I got it out and tried it again.

One night my mother and father took me to the Maryland Academy of Science so I could get a chance to look through their telescope at Jupiter. Well, I almost got a chance to look through it. When I got up to the eyepiece the clouds moved in. We waited for about a half an hour, but the clouds stayed and we had to go home.

Christmas was an exciting time. The electric trains were set out on a platform that was about 6' square and raised six inches off the floor. It was painted green to represent grass. A Christmas tree, all decorated with the electric lights and balls and tinsel was in the middle of the platform. The presents were off to the side and I found one that had my name on it. I eagerly tore away the bright Christmas paper and discovered a small telescope inside. The telescope had about one inch aperture. It had about seven power. I know this because I still have it and I later learned how to measure its magnifying power. In these times of the Great Depression, my father had most likely bought the telescope at a pawnshop and cleaned it up. He had made a leather case for it. He had also made a tripod. It was all that I wanted. It whetted my interest in astronomy for many years.

One of the nice things about Christmas was going to visit friends' houses and seeing all the neat things they got. I remember that one of my friends had received a lead-casting machine. This had various dies that would make lead soldiers in various battle positions. I thought this was great. I wanted one too, but I never did get one. However, I think that it encouraged my interest in melting and casting lead, which I soon began to do.

Another thing I remember about Christmas is going to visit the displays of electric trains at firehouses. I remember that one of the best ones was at the firehouse on Gay Street. They had the trains up on a platform along one side of the firehouse. The platform must have been about the length of a fire engine and about as deep as a fire engine is wide. They had all kinds of trains running on different tracks, steam engines, diesel electrics, and electric locomotives. But I remember that they had a monorail train. I had never seen one of these before even as a model. Wow!

I was also interested in chemistry and one Christmas I got a chemical set. It had a booklet that described how to do all sorts of experiments with the chemicals in the set and also some with household chemicals. The following year I got an even larger set. I doubt that chemical sets like those are available today because of concerns about hazards. But I sure had fun. One of the things I pursued was blowing glass. Initially, this was just making bends in tubing. But then I also made little bubbles at the end of the tubing by melting and blowing.

I went down to my public library branch and took out a college-level textbook on chemistry. The book had color pictures of precipitates and descriptions of all kinds of chemical reactions. I could only keep the book out for two weeks. At the end of this time, I went back and renewed it for another two weeks. Then I would wait a week and take it out again for another two weeks. And so forth. I never read it through from start to finish. I couldn't handle some of the material. I would skip around, reading what I liked. The librarian was very curious about my interests in the college-level textbook. I learned what reacted with what, and what didn't react with what. Years later, after encountering students that had recent courses in chemistry that stressed theory and problems, I realized that they didn't know what would react with what, etc.

Circa Age 15

Lee, my boyhood friend from next door, and I took the streetcar down to the Maryland Academy of Science one evening to look through their telescope. We arrived there about 7:00 p.m. in the evening when they opened. After considerable discussion with a man at the door, we were not allowed to enter because we were not accompanied by an adult. That was their rule and he was not about to make an exception. Dejectedly, we went back home by streetcar again. I never did get to look through their 12-inch telescope. I can now understand their position in not wanting to let unaccompanied kids in, but I subsequently became an astronomer and they didn't help that. It still is a sore point.

My interest in astronomy sort of waned following the trip down to the Maryland Academy of Science and I got interested in ham radio. I built a shortwave receiver and tuned into the ham bands. I studied the Morse code and I practiced copying the messages being sent between hams. Gradually, I built up my speed in copying but it was a struggle. As in learning to type, one reaches plateaus at certain speeds. The required speed for a license was to be able to copy and send Morse code at 13 words per minute. With just about everyone, there is a very firm plateau at about eight words per minute. In June 1940, I was ready not only to copy 13 words per minute but also to take a written examination about ham radio theory and regulations.

The examinations were given in a small building on the other side of Fort Sreet from Fort McHenry,

Baltimore, Maryland. The reason the FCC had its office on the waterfront was that they were called upon to inspect marine radios.

My father dropped me off at the FCC office at about 8:30 on a Saturday morning in July. I went inside and a sign directed me to the second floor. There I met a lady clacking away on a typewriter. She stopped in a moment and I nervously told her what I wanted. She checked over my documents, I had to have personal identification and proof of citizenship, and then she asked me to be seated and to wait for the examiner. In a short while, he came across the room from where he was working and asked me to follow him. He gave me the written examination to take. It was an essay test as I had expected. The questions, though, were from among those that had been published. I had studied them well and passed the test with no problem. Then came the Morse code test, the most dreaded part was copying code at 13 words per minute. But apparently I did OK for he then asked me to send some text using the telegraph key. I did this, and he said I passed. Whoopee! I went home on the streetcar, but I was floating on air.

Because the FCC was backlogged with all sorts of merchant marine applications in 1940 and the necessity to checkout the citizenship of applicants, it was not until December 13, 1940 that I got my license in the mail. My call letters were W3JBQ, not a good call for sending in Morse code. Oh well, I was tickled. I immediately called up my friend, John Cann, W3IEM, for a schedule on the radio. This was my first contact. John was one of my "elmers". An elmer is a ham who helps others to get started in ham radio. Another of my elmers was John Carter, W3ELO. He was about six years older than I and was my brother's pal. During the following year, or actually up to December 7, 1941, I had many more than 1000 contacts. According to my log, which I still have, I contacted all 48 states and also the Canal Zone. In this pre-war era, Americans were not allowed to contact any foreign countries except for U.S. territories. In fact, in 1940 most amateurs in foreign countries were not allowed on the air. On that infamous Sunday morning in 1941, there were radio announcements from the American Radio Relay League that our licenses were suspended by the FCC and all ham activity was to cease.

One of my friends, T. King McCubbin, Jr., whom I called King, took the tests for his ham license several months before I did, but because his birth certificate said only "McCubbin boy", his application was initially returned and he had to get his christening certificate to prove his citizenship. About a week after I got my license, King called me up and arranged to schedule a contact on the radio. The issuance of his license had been delayed until he had satisfactory proof of his citizenship. His call letters were W3JBZ. They didn't issue very many licenses in that week.

In the summer, my parents, Bob and I often took vacations at Ocean City, Maryland, which is on the eastern shore (on the other side of the Chesapeake Bay from Baltimore, Maryland). To get there in those days before the Bay Bridge was built, we had to drive around the bay or else we could go by ferry across the bay. My father usually chose to drive around rather than pay the ferry fee and also to have to endure the wait. I liked going on the ferry because they were sidewheel paddle steamboats. Some had large seesaw devices on the uppermost deck. This device connected on one side to the piston of the large steam cylinder and on the other side it connected to the crankshaft that drove the paddle wheels.

On one such vacation, I felt very ill at the end of it. I was running a high fever and we took the ferry home. When we got home, my father called Dr. Wantz. He said that he thought I had malaria. I don't recall a blood smear ever being done to look for parasites, but I didn't think that the diagnosis of malaria was reasonable. Much later on, I read about there being such a thing as non-paralytic polio. I understand now that some authorities say that 80 percent of the population has had polio at some time or other. I think it is quite possible that is what I had.

In the eighth grade of junior high school, I applied to get into the ninth grade of the high school, Baltimore Polytechnic Institute, which was actually part of the public school system. This would have put me into the A course, whose curriculum included calculus. Unfortunately, I was not able to get into the A course because I did not have a 75 percent grade in all subjects. I only had 70 percent grade in history so I had to settle for the B course, which didn't transfer me until the 10th grade.

I really enjoyed going to Poly. I was turned on by the courses in chemistry, physics, electricity and magnetism, even steam engineering. Some of the math courses were tedious because calculations had to be exactly correct. I had to remember to always multiply before dividing in order to maintain accuracy to whatever the number of decimal places that were required. Trigonometry was especially hard because of the difficulty of adding up a column of five digit logarithm numbers accurately.

We had a number of laboratory courses. There were laboratory courses for chemistry, physics and for electricity. And there was also a laboratory course that went along with steam engineering. This class was held down in the basement of the west wing where a rather large steam engine powered a D.C. generator that produced electricity for the west wing. They started the generator at 8:00 a.m. in the morning and shut it down at 2: 30 p.m. when school was out. During the rest of the time, the west wing was switched over to commercial A.C. power.

In this laboratory course, we measured the strength of steel, calibrated pressure gauges, measured the heat value of coal, determined the horsepower put out by the steam engine, and performed other interesting tests. At the end of this course, we spent one whole day running the steam engine and the boiler. Each class got a grade on how they performed. There were all kinds of mistakes that students could make and for each mistake points were taken off of the class score. The class with the best score got five points added to each student's grade. A fearful mistake was turning the valve the wrong way and overfilling the large vat of water that was weighed before the water went into the boilers. There was much hurry to keep up with the boilers' requirements.

We also had a class work course in steam engineering, which was given by Helm Rogers. I thought I did well in steam engineering. Other students were always asking me how to work various problems. But when the final exam came around, I apparently didn't do very well as I got a poor grade.

At the end of each semester, we had two-hour examinations in each subject. Two of these examinations were given each morning and after about 1:00 p.m. we were free to go home and study for the next day's exams.

During one set of the examinations, I noticed that I was having terrible head-aches. I don't know now whether this was coincidental in time or not, but my father had brought me some cadmium wire and I became busy in trying to make an alloy of cadmium and lead. They didn't seem to mix and so I was heating the lead to high temperatures. This was down in my basement where the ventilation was poor. I presume now that these were concurrent and my headaches were from metal poisoning.

The ham radio club, which of course I joined, had a club room that was off of the drafting room in which Mr. Rogers taught. The club room was in the west wing. We had radio equipment that used transformers to step up the commercial A.C. power to voltages used by vacuum tubes. Well, it's not hard to imagine that some student would forget to turn off the equipment before going home at the end of the day. Next morning when the power switched over to D.C. power at 8 a.m., the transformers, which do not like D.C. power, would burn out. Pretty soon Mr. Rogers' drafting room would fill with acrid smoke. I believe this happened twice.

The radio club did another thing that also made Mr. Rogers unhappy. Each June on one weekend, amateur radio operators go out into the field and set up portable equipment to help themselves prepare for emergency situations. These outings are usually organized by clubs. The Poly radio club went on such an outing. To generate electricity, we borrowed a generator from the electricity laboratory. One of the students had an old gas-powered washing machine motor. A vee belt connected pulleys on the generator and the motor. To hold these together, we mounted them on a board that someone found in our clubroom. Because the board was too long, it was sawed off at a suitable length. It turned out that this board was a leaf from Mr. Rogers' dining room table. He had brought it in to refinish it in the wood shop. It was mahogany. The radio club had to pay for a new leaf for Mr. Rogers out of the club treasury. After that the radio club was asked to move to another room in the central wing of the school where A.C. power was supplied all of the time.

A friend of mine, who was also a ham, lived out on a rural road beyond Towson, Maryland. He had no phone because telephone lines had not extended along his rural road. One night a bad car accident happened in front of his house. He got hold of me on the radio and asked me to call the Towson police and an ambulance. It was a long-distance call, which was expensive in those days. Anyhow, I looked up the Towson police number and told them about the accident. They wanted to know how it was that I was reporting an accident that was many miles away from me. I had a hard time convincing them that I made this contact through ham radio and that I wasn't making a joke. Finally they agreed to send an officer out to investigate and to send an ambulance. My friend later told me that the injured people, who were taken to the hospital, were okay.

After the war started, amateurs got interested in all sorts of electronic things that didn't involve radio. I built a device to talk over the light beam from a flashlight. This would work up to a couple hundred feet. John Cann and I constructed equipment to talk over the power lines using a very low frequency. I believe that we sent Morse code over the distance between our houses, which was about three-quarters of a mile. The connection was very noisy, but we succeeded in communicating.

John got inducted into the army and went off to communications school. I became interested in photography and had a 35-mm camera. My father and I built a dark room in the basement where I began developing film and enlarging pictures. This got me into all kinds of new chemicals.

Bob, who had always been interested in airplanes, had enlisted so he could get into the Air Corps. He was accepted into this and was shipped off to Akron, Ohio for basic training. During the summer, after my highschool graduation, Mom, Dad, and I went by train to visit Bob in Akron. This was a new experience for me, for I had never ridden in a Pullman car before. I had the upper bunk. I don't think I slept very well.

Off to War

Booommm!

An artillery shell exploded about three feet from our foxhole. It was October, 1944, and I was in Alsace-Lorraine near Nancy in France. Our company had just gone into combat that day, making it my first time. We climbed up a hill and were told to dig in. My buddy, Paul, and I dug a foxhole. Paul said he had seen a sheet of armor plate that apparently had come off a half-track personnel carrier. We carried this piece of steel, which was about 2 feet by 4 feet, to our foxhole and placed it over top and covered it over with the dirt from the foxhole. We put one of our ground covers over the opening because it looked like it would rain.

The ground cover was riddled with holes from the shrapnel of the shell. Almost immediately, it began to rain. It became quiet. I looked out around us and in the gray glow of the mist in the ending twilight I thought that the cedar trees were enemy soldiers approaching us. I thought I saw the cedars move and so I threw several hand grenades at them. I was scared. I'm sure Paul was too.

When I woke up next morning on the battlefield, Paul was missing. I asked my platoon sergeant where he'd gone. The platoon sergeant said he was shell-shocked and he had gone back to the medical aid tent. I never saw him again.

I was not psyched out for what was happening in combat, especially the artillery shells. I was terrified, but I wasn't going to run away. I was too ingrained with patriotism and doing the right thing. That is, not being a deserter and being court-martialed. Let me review what my training had been since high school.

I got a letter in August following my graduation from high school. The letter began "Greetings!" It was my draft notice to report in September. First, I got a physical. This was the first time I ever had blood drawn from a vein. I think I nearly fainted. I guess I passed the physical because I was classified as 1A. Then I was off to Fort Meade. I was issued uniforms and all sorts of gear. The stuff filled a barracks bag, which I think weighed a hundred pounds. I lugged it to the barracks where a sergeant showed us how to make up bunks according to Army specifications. I remember breakfast the next morning. The combination of coffee, which I don't believe I ever had before, and the greasy sausage and eggs, nearly turned my stomach. After a short stay there, we were off by train to Fort Jackson, South Carolina for basic training. I was very lonely. I survived on weekly letters from my Dad and occasional letters from Bob, who was now an Air Corps pilot.

At the end of basic training, we were given the Army General Classification Test, which I think is much like an IQ test. Anyhow, I scored 133, which I gather is pretty good. I had been accepted into the ASTP, which stood for the Army Specialized Training Program and that meant that I would be off to college after my basic training. I was off to the University of Maine. It was now December, and brother, was it cold. There was a lot of snow, and one morning the temperature was 24° below zero. One very sad thing happened while I was there. One of the dormitories burned down in the middle of the night. One of my friends, I'll call him Svensen - he was from Minnesota - escaped from the dormitory unscathed. But his friend in the upper bunk wasn't so lucky. Svensen woke him up and was sure he was awake for he was putting on his shoes, but he didn't seem to make it out of the fire. Afterwards, my friend would have nightmares about it and had a phobia about smoke.

I did pretty well in my course work, I believe I got an 'A' in physics and an 'A' in geography. But then I already knew a lot of the geography from my interest in ham radio. I don't remember any of the other courses. The Army Specialized Training Program came to an end in April 1945 because the army needed soldiers for the invasion of Europe. We were to be shipped to the 26th Infantry Division, which was on maneuvers in Kentucky. We had a few days before we were going to be shipped out so I got a textbook on Calculus from the library. In 93 hours total elapsed time, I studied the entire part on differential Calculus and worked every problem. Then I went into Bangor and bought a textbook on Calculus to take with me to Kentucky.

We were then off on a troop train. The train had troop cars that slept soldiers crosswise on the car and three bunks high. I believe they had a baggage car that was converted into a kitchen. We took our mess kits and went through a serving line to get our meals. And they had the usual three garbage cans to wash our mess kits.

In Kentucky, we were billeted in a camp that had 9 ft. square tents, which I believe slept six men. We had the the usual Red Army force which fought the Blue Army force using blanks. After about two weeks in Kentucky, the 26th Infantry Division moved to Fort Benning, Georgia. The division had now been brought up to full strength (26,000 men) and we continued training there. We made frequent trips out to the rifle range and for the first time we were issued Garrand rifles which, in army technology, were known as M1s.

Of course, some of the soldiers in the Division had been there ever since it was part of the Massachusetts National Guard. Our platoon sergeant was not well educated and spoke with a drawl. This made for some mistrust between educated soldiers who came from the ASTP and this sergeant. One day the sergeant was trying to teach us about the sights on the M1 rifle and he kept referring to the "ampitire" (meaning aperture). Each time he said it we would begin giggling. Finally, the lieutenant told us to keep our mouths shut or we would be put on KP duty.

The lieutenant for our platoon was really a nice person. Lieutenant Wray had been in the regular army before the war. In other words, he was in the U.S. Army and not the Army of the United States, which draftees were in. He must have been about 50 at the time and the story was that he had worked his way up through the ranks. He kept his shoes polished like a mirror and they were dark brown rather than being a lighter brown as ours were. Also, his uniform was ironed and neat. But most important of all, I felt that he was a leader because he set good examples for people to follow rather than using discipline to enforce regulations.

I think every military outfit has a misfit. In our company this was Burlingame. It was customary that we would have an inspection of rifles after we returned from the rifle range to see if we had cleaned the rifle. The lieutenant would come in front of each soldier in turn as we stood in formation. As the lieutenant came in front of us, we did a "present arms", which meant we brought the rifle from resting with its butt on the ground to a 45 degree position in front of us and at the same time pulled the bolt back so that the lieutenant could take the rifle from us and look down the barrel. As Burlingame pulled the bolt back, a live round popped out of the gun. Of course, Burlingame got a week or more of KP duty.

We were frequently going out to the rifle range. I qualified as marksman, which was part of the requirements for the Expert Infantry Badge. Some of the other requirements were various timed hikes with rifle and full field pack. We had to do 4 miles in 50 minutes, 9 miles in 2 hours, and 25 miles in 8 hours. We also had to complete obstacle courses, but it was worth it for the Expert Infantry Badge added $5 to the $21 monthly pay. One course we had was to crawl across a field with machine-gun fire going over our heads. This course had explosions going off in the middle of the field to simulate artillery shells, but I later came to realize that this was not like the real thing. If you kept your butt down and avoided the places where the charges were, you were pretty certain to get across the field safely. That certainly is different from thinking you might lose your life crossing the field. I wasn't prepared for the misery either.

The weather became really rainy and cold and I no longer had a buddy. One night, it was raining hard and our access road had been cut off by the Germans. The result of this was that we had no food. I dug a foxhole, but it filled up with water. I found a tree with some hard apples on it. I ate maybe one but was afraid of what they might do to me. I was miserable. I began to think about what kind of a wound I would be able to live with. I didn't want to be blind. But I knew that I wanted to become a scientist and I could put up with a lot of disability.

Everything was so muddy. When walking along roads, my boots would get so caked up with mud that I could hardly lift them up. I would try to scrape them off on any object, like a log, but they would get caked up almost immediately. It was tough going, and it was miserable. One of the things that we were told was that if we got trench foot and had to be put in the hospital that we could be court martialed. We were always supposed to have a pair of dry socks. But that hardly seemed possible considering that it was raining every day.

One day, this may have been right after we were cut off, we moved from one place to another by truck. I believe we moved four times, digging in at each place. This is a technique to confuse the enemy into believing that we were moving into a sector with considerable strength. It was hard work digging all those foxholes. And now I had a bad cold.

Thwuummp! I had seen the flash of an artillery shell about 30 feet to my right. Instantly, I felt a searing pain in my left calf. I fell to the ground, which is where I should have been in the first place. Incoming artillery shells usually whistle and you can tell by the Doppler shift how far away from you that they will land. But you hear very little before one lands next to you.

We had been moving up a hill toward a town that was at the top. Now I would have to take care of my wound. I took off my legging and pulled up my pants leg

40

exposing a wound that was about the size of a half dollar on the inner side of the left calf. I got out the packet of sulfanilamide powder, which we all carried in a first-aid kit. I applied the powder and put on a bandage. I lay there for quite awhile because I would need help getting up the hill. Finally, one of my fellow soldiers came by and helped me struggle up the hill. We found a building in the town where I could get into the basement. We figured this was safer if there was more shelling. This could have been a bad move as I found out later. My friend had to go on and catch up to the company so he left me to wait for help.

After about an hour, I heard voices outside and called to them. They asked me to come out. I told them that I wasn't able to. They demanded that I should come out. My calf had swollen and had become very painful. After I told them that I was badly wounded one of them came in and helped me up the stairs and out of the building. I was glad that they didn't throw in a hand grenade. That's why being in the basement was a bad idea. Soon, an ambulance came and picked me up and transported me to a front-line hospital in Nancy.

The piece of shrapnel had penetrated all the way across my calf and lay close to the surface on the other side. So they took it out from the other side. My leg became fairly infected and I believe I got one of the very first shots of penicillin. My cold was really bad and they gave me a swig of G.I. gin (codeine-terpen hydrate in 40 percent alcohol). I was feeling a lot better the next day and it was Thanksgiving. I was in the hospital just in time for a Thanksgiving turkey dinner.

After staying here for a few days, I was moved back by train to a hospital in Cherbourg. I believe that I stayed there until after Christmas. Then I went back to a rehabilitation hospital near Cambridge, England. The doctors there discovered two things about my wound. I could not bend my foot up as far as my other foot. I also had a loss of feeling on the top of my foot. One doctor went around my foot with a pin pricking it to find out where I could feel the prick and where I couldn't and he marked this with a pen. When he was finished, he had outlined an area that included most of the top of my foot. Obviously, a nerve had been damaged as a result of the wound and the muscle was greatly damaged which limited my foot motion.

By April, 1945, I had fully recovered and they sent me back to my company of the 26th Division. By this time, my company had been to the Battle of the Bulge, and the Division was part of Patton's Third Army. The remaining part of the war involved chasing the retreating Germans until they capitulated. I ended up in Czechoslovakia. In about a month's time, we pulled back across the Danube River into Austria because it had been decided that Czechoslovakia would be in the Russian Zone. It was here that I received devastating news from my mother. My brother, Bob, who was pilot of a B-17 that was based in Italy, was shot down over Linz, Austria. At that point, he was only listed as missing, but he was later reported as deceased. I remembered seeing a bomber come crashing about a mile away when we were near Linz, Austria. But that was a B-24, not a B-17.

I've missed Bob. I wonder what a difference he would have made in my life. After the war was over, his fiancee came to visit my mother and father. I think she wanted to check me out because she told me that Bob and I were as different as night and day.

Getting Educated

The scene was the office of the head of the math department, Johns Hopkins University. The office was tiny but it did have a nice view looking out to a spacious green lawn that led down to Charles Street, the central north-south street of Baltimore. It was January, 1946, and I had been discharged from the army in December. My father went with me when I registered. He wanted to help me get into Johns Hopkins at the last moment before classes started. He wanted me to register in engineering, but I was adamant that I wanted to study physics, which of course was in the School of Arts and Sciences.

WMS: "Sir, I am hoping that you will approve granting me credit for elementary calculus. Although I have not had any formal training in calculus, I have studied it on my own and I've worked every problem in the textbook by Osgood. This I did at the end of my Army Specialized Training Program during and after my assignment at the University of Maine. I really understand calculus quite well."

Dr. Rich Darkmatter: "I'm sorry, but you will have to talk with Mr. Max Minn. He is your assigned instructor for the course. There is nothing that I can do without his approval." (I tried to track down Mr. Minn, but he seemed not to be available. It was now just before the first class and I confronted Mr. Minn in the classroom.)

WMS: "Mr. Minn., I'm hoping that you'll grant me credit for differential calculus. I've studied the book by Osgood and I've worked every problem in the book. I really know calculus quite well."

Mr. Minn: "If that is the book that you have studied, you do not understand the fundamental basis for the calculus. I'm sorry, but you will have to take this course in order to proceed with your studies."

So for the rest of the course I sat in the back of the room and was completely bored. I brought books to study on amateur radio antennas. Much later, I wished I had spent my time studying differential equations, which would have been my next step in the study of math. Actually, if I'd been well advised, I would have learned that this was the next step. But I didn't know this at the time. During the summer break, I got a book on the calculus of variations, which is an interesting topic, but it is not necessary to study this in the progression of mathematics.

I did well in science classes such as chemistry and physics. Of course, I was majoring in physics, so I was expected to do well in these. I did only fair in English writing and languages such as German. My downfall, again, was in history. Also, I didn't do well in Political Science. Now there is an oxymoron. And of course, I did pretty well in mathematics.

I spent a lot of my free time in the Radio Club, and I was president of that for several years. The call sign for the club was W3GQF. The radio club doesn't seem to exist anymore. The interests of students seems to have changed over the years.

My tuition and a stipend was paid for by the G.I. Bill of Rights. I was living with my parents and so I paid them rent. Much of the rest of the money I invested in ham radio equipment. I spent a lot of time on the air. I contacted a number of foreign countries. I also got interested in microwaves and, with the help of the Radio Club, made some contacts on 3-cm wavelength, considered very short at the time. This was possible using parts from war surplus radar equipment.

During this period, I took up several projects constructing optical instruments with help from Edmund Salvage Co. (now Edmund Scientific Co.). They supplied many war-surplus optical gadgets. I bought some glass prisms and lenses from them and designed and built a photographic spectrograph (a device for recording the component colors of light). Edmund had a contest that was based on gadgets built with their stuff and so I wrote up a report on the spectrograph. I won five dollars of merchandise.

With this money, I bought a kit to make an astronomical telescope mirror. Making the mirror required shoving one 8-inch diameter piece of plate glass over a similar one which is affixed to the top of a barrel, all the while walking around the barrel so that no particular direction is favored. This is done with finer and finer grades of grinding grits and water in between and then finishing with rouge polish.

The mirror must be tested, of course. There is an indoor test that can be done, but I couldn't resist the temptation to try it outdoors. I had no mounting for the telescope. I took the mirror outside one evening as the moon was rising. By propping the mirror up in the grass alongside the roadway and lying in the gutter while holding an eyepiece up to my eye, I could get a good view of the moon. A car came along and the driver stopped. Apparently, he thought I might be drunk.

Toward the end of my senior year, I applied for admission into the Graduate School to study Physics. I also applied for a job with Prof. John Strong in the physics department. His field was optics and especially infrared optics. My friend, King McCubbin, already worked for him as a graduate student. King was a year ahead of me through college. This was really because he got into the A course at Baltimore Polytechnic Institute, while I only got into the B course. It all went back to my doing poorly in history in junior high school. The sins of my past caught up with me.

I was very naive as this was the only graduate school to which I applied. It never occurred to me that I might be turned down. But apparently, I had made an impression on John Strong in my interview. He wanted to know about my hobbies. I was accepted into graduate school and of course, I was hired by Strong as a graduate assistant. Strong assigned me to work with my friend King McCubbin. It was Strong's policy to have new students work for older students while they were preparing for their thesis dissertations. King did his thesis on far infrared spectroscopy. Far infrared means wavelengths of the order of 0.1 to 1 millimeter. These are just like light waves but are just short of radio wavelengths.

My first scientific paper was published with King as the first author. Together, we published several papers on the far infrared. I also worked on other things that gave me papers on several other subjects. One project involved observing the sun at 1-mm wavelength, which had never been done before. This resulted in a paper in the Physical

Review Letters, a prestigious journal. One of my friends suggested that I paste together a number my papers and submit this as a thesis. But I didn't seriously consider this.

To become a candidate for the Ph.D. in physics, a student had to pass five oral examinations in various topics in physics. Each of these oral examinations was given by an assigned member of the physics faculty. If a student failed one of these examinations, he or she could petition to take the examination one more time. Students who failed the second time were out of the Department. The five examinations were capped with a final examination by the entire physics faculty.

My first oral examination was given by Professor Bearden and was to be in modern physics. In one of the questions, he asked me for details of an experiment that tested the atomic nature of matter. I didn't do very well in recalling and explaining the significance of this experiment. He flunked me on the exam. He also told me that I would never become a successful scientist.

I was very dejected and became very depressed. I considered committing suicide - I could not become a scientist. I considered that I should jump from the balcony on the fifth floor of the physics building and land on a walkway into the building. Eventually I realized that this would not accomplish anything except to destroy myself. I studied modern physics very hard and petitioned to take the exam again. I passed this the second time.

I passed the other four exams and then applied to take the final examination, which would be at least a two hour oral exam. During this exam, Professor Bearden asked me the same question that he had flunked me on before. I answered it in a great amount of detail, so much so that they had to stop me so that they could go on to some other question. At the end of the examination, they asked other professors in the room if they would like to ask me any questions. A professor in theoretical physics asked me it if it was possible to detect gravitational waves from double stars. I told him flatly that I didn't know whether this was possible. I knew I had passed the exam.

John Strong called me into his office one day. He made a proposal that I should accompany him out to Palomar Observatory and work with him on acquiring infrared spectra of planets. This could then be the subject for my thesis. He wrote to the director of Palomar. The reply suggested that we first try our equipment at the 100-inch telescope on Mount Wilson. So in the summer of 1952, I went to Mt. Wilson with John Strong. We rode out to Pasadena, California on The Capitol Limited and The Chief. Strong didn't like flying. Also, he didn't like The Super Chief because it was too bumpy because it went faster.

We took an instrument that had been dubbed the "big monster." It was an infrared spectrograph that Strong had designed and made for the 200-inch telescope at Palomar. The alignment of planets was not very good in 1952, though we did get good spectra of Mercury. The main thing we learned was how to proceed with next year at Palomar. We went back to Hopkins and I worked on improving the optics of the "big monster." I managed to improve the transmission of light through the spectrograph from 10% to 75%, which is where it should have been.

In my free time, I worked on improving my skills at blowing glass. I made some little glasses for after dinner liqueurs. I was spending some hours each day in a room that had no windows. An inspector from the Baltimore City Health Department came to measure the amount of mercury vapor in the air in various laboratories at Hopkins. He discovered that the room where I was working had unusually high values of mercury vapor. There was asphalt tile on the floor and it seems that mercury had gotten into the cracks between the tiles. The only way to clean this up was to tear up the tile on the floor.

Two of my friends, let's call them Bill and Chad, also worked for John Strong. They used infrared equipment that was on the fifth floor of Rowland Hall. The equipment required dry ice for cooling its infrared detector. Dry ice was stored in the sub-basement. They had a wooden box with a handle like a suitcase to carry the dry ice up to the fifth floor. They were given special permission to use the elevator to carry the dry ice up to their workroom but not to carry the box back down. One evening, after Bill and Chad had gone home, I took the box down to the shop and removed the screws that held the bottom on to the box. The sides of the box were about 5/8 inches thick. I got a 3/8 inch drill and drilled about 30 holes, each about 6 in. deep. I then cast 30 lead slugs, each 3/8 in. diameter and 6 in. long. Then every evening after Bill and Chad had gone home I would add one of these lead slugs to the box.

Initially, the box weighed a couple of pounds. By the time that all of the slugs were added, its weight had increased to 15 pounds. Bill and Chad would take the box from their office on the second floor down to the sub-basement, fill it with dry ice, take the box up the elevator to the fifth floor, and at the end of the day they would carry the empty box down the stairs and hallways to their office. Before I started putting lead slugs into the box, they would swing it back and forth as they strode along.

By the time that the box approached 15 pounds, they would carry it as a dead weight and put it down if they stopped to talk to someone on the way. Nearly everyone in Rowland Hall learned what was going on, but no one spilled the beans to Bill and Chad. It wasn't until one day when they visited one of their chemistry buddies in another building that the truth dawned on them. Their buddy asked them who this practical joke was being played on over in Rowland Hall. John Strong was much impressed with my shop work on the box because I had drilled all of these holes without having the drill come out through the other side of the box. This was a big risk I took, but it all worked out.

My father and I made a mercury barometer. This led me to try to make another instrument that was also a barometer of sorts. It was supposed to measure the rate of change of the barometric pressure, and it, too, used mercury. I believe it would have been a new invention, but it didn't work and I never did anything further with it. So I had various exposures to mercury. I also had exposure to other chemicals. I used uranium metal to make a getter (a material that maintains the vacuum in a closed system like a vacuum tube). I also had some exposure to thorium, which is much more radioactive than uranium. I also utilized thallium chloride and bromide and selenium and tellurium metals.

The following year I finished my thesis, which was titled "Temperatures and Spectra of Venus." I received my doctorate degree in October 1953. I stayed on at Hopkins for one year with a post-doctorate appointment.

Girls, Kids, and Mars

At the end of my one-year postdoctoral at Hopkins, I received a letter from Harvard College Observatory inviting me to apply for the position of lecturer and research associate. Apparently, I had an impressive recommendation from John Strong. It seemed that everyone, even my parents, knew about my pending appointment before I did. Anyhow, I accepted the appointment and moved to Cambridge, Massachusetts in late summer of 1954. This was just in time for Hurricane Carol. My parents went up with me to help me get settled. Carol struck while we were on a bus tour of Boston. At the end of the tour, trees were coming down and department store windows were being broken and mannequins were flying down the street. When we got back to Cambridge, a church steeple was rocking back and forth and threatening to come down. It didn't, but it remained canted at a peculiar angle. I rented an apartment at 49 Irving Street. It was not a very nice apartment but I could be comfortable in it. Besides, it had a gas refrigerator that was still working despite the power outage from the storm. Mom and Dad left the next day, and I reported to work at Harvard.

With Dr. Gerhard Miczaika, I got involved in refurbishing the 24-inch and 61-inch Harvard telescopes. One of the things I had experience in was aluminizing telescope mirrors. John Strong was the inventor of this process and I gained a lot of experience from him. Miczaika and I also got involved in writing a book for the Harvard College Observatory series on astronomy. We called the book "Tools of the Astronomer," and it dealt with modern telescopes and the equipment used on them.

I had never before been interested in pursuing women. But now I found one that interested me. She was a graduate student at Harvard. Today, it would be a no-no for an instructor to pursue a graduate student, but then there didn't seem to be anything wrong with that. In the end, this relationship didn't work out.

I kept on pursuing my research interests (and women). I wanted to find something to do that would be outstanding and to make a name for myself. There was a reason that Mars was called the red and green planet. The green was supposed to be vegetation. The vegetation ought to have absorption bands in the vicinity of 3.5 microns wavelength (this is in the infrared). Plant leaves should absorb at this wavelength because of the vibration of the hydrogen atoms against the adjacent carbon atoms. W. W. Coblentz (an infrared physicist who was formerly with the U.S. Bureau of Standards) had shown such an absorption by vegetation in one of his monographs. So I built equipment to find this absorption on Mars. I would use this on the 61-inch telescope, which was the largest telescope available to me for such an uncertain project. The amount of infrared signal from Mars was very weak. I had to spend many hours observing the wavelengths of the feature over and over and even then I had to use a statistical analysis to test if the absorption feature was present. In the end, I believed I had a statistically significant result showing that there was vegetation on Mars. I published the result in the *Astrophysical Journal.*

Despite this success, I don't think that I was very productive at Harvard. I didn't have many colleagues who were doing the type of research that I was interested in. I now realize that what was lacking was the infrastructure to support my type of front-line research. I didn't have anyone to talk to on a regular basis about physical studies of planets. At the end of three years there, I realized that I was not accomplishing very much. So I wrote a letter to the director of Lowell Observatory inquiring about a position with the Observatory. In due course, I received a letter back from the sole trustee of the Observatory, Roger L. Putnam, offering me the position of Astronomer. On the strength of this, I bought a new car, a Chevy station wagon. In June, 1957, I packed all my belongings into the station wagon and headed west for Flagstaff, Arizona. I had been in Flagstaff several times before, in 1952 and 1953 for meetings of the International Mars Committee.

I already knew most of the people at Lowell and I fit in well with them. I enjoyed the informality of getting shop work done and being able to order equipment without the hassle of finding competitive bids unless required by the contract. Through contacts that I made with the Air Force Cambridge Research Laboratory when at Harvard, I was able to get a contract with them for some of my research at Lowell. I also applied for, and got, a grant from the National Science Foundation to purchase equipment for infrared research on the planets. I built equipment to measure temperatures of planets, work that followed up on my thesis. I also built equipment to extend the previous observations of the vegetation bands on Mars. (By the way, these became known as the Sinton bands). After building new and better equipment than I had at Harvard, I applied for observing time on the 200-inch Palomar telescope. I guess I made a good case as they granted me the time. It was unusual to grant time to an outsider to do work on planets on the world's largest telescope. I obtained what I thought was very convincing spectra showing the 3.5-micron bands. They seemed to be stronger in the green areas of Mars than in the red areas. I was elated, it seemed to be a real discovery. I wrote up the paper for *Science Journal.* Before sending it off, I agonized over whether something was wrong with the data, but I could not figure out what was wrong so I sent it off.

Dr. Earl C. Slipher, who had become acting director of Lowell after the resignation of the previous director, had done years of research photographing Mars. He needed an assistant to help him with analyzing the photographs. A graduate of Carleton College, Miss Marjorie Korner came to Lowell for the position. It wasn't long before we were dating. In June, 1960, we were married. Our wedding reception was held in the rotunda of the Lowell Observatory. Marge and I had three boys, Bob, David and Alan. Raising my boys was lots of fun. My life was, and still is, enriched by my boys. They have also given me a tremendous amount of pride.

The time that I was at Lowell Observatory was the most productive time in my career. But now, Roger Putnam told Marge not to make it to too easy for me. I'm not sure what he meant. After having our first two boys, Marge wanted to come back to work for me. John Hall, the director of Lowell, told us that the Observatory had an anti-nepotism policy and that Marge could not work for me.

In 1964, I received a letter from Dr. Donald Rea. He said that he had some serious questions concerning the possibility that the Sinton bands were produced by heavy water molecules in the Earth's atmosphere since two of the wavelengths of the three bands corresponded exactly with absorption dips caused by the heavy water molecule, HDO. He asked whether he and an associate, Dr. Kenneth Watson, could come and look at my data. I said yes, and that he was welcome to. I think it was a fortunate thing that I did have the data looked at independently from me. They found out that there was a flaw in my results in that the comparison solar spectrum was taken in the daytime several hours after the Mars spectra were obtained. This was a necessity because I was only given telescope time in the early morning hours and there was not time to do a nearly simultaneous observation of lunar spectra. They found that on the day that I had done the solar spectra, it was considerably drier than the nights when the Mars spectra were taken. Hence, the Mars spectrum, after being corrected by division by the solar spectrum, showed apparent absorptions at the wavelengths of the HDO bands. The third band and the apparent prevalence of the absorption in green areas is still not explained. It is surprising that that spectra of Mars in this region, that is 3.5 microns, have not been obtained since, even with much better equipment today and with capability for spacecraft observations. Some recent ground-based work has shown some indication of vegetation, but direct in situ observations from the Viking spacecraft showed nothing that looked like organic molecules, much less vegetation.

I Choose To Live

13,800 Feet

"Come along boys and listen to my tale,

I 'll tell you 'bout my troubles on the Mauna Kea trail.

Come a Ki Yi Yippie, Yippie Yea, Yippie Yea.

Come a Ki Yi Yippie, Yippie Yea".

Full text of song in appendix B

    In the spring of 1965, I received a letter from Dr. John Jefferies, the director of the Haleakala Observatory, which was part of the Hawaii Institute of Geophysics of the University of Hawaii. He told me that he had a contract from NASA to build an 84-inch telescope on either Haleakala or on Mauna Kea. Haleakala is a 10,000-foot mountain on Maui and Mauna Kea is a nearly 14,000-foot mountain on the Island of Hawaii. I was already acquainted with these mountains from a report that was given by a meteorologist at one of the Mars Committee meetings. He reported that the amount of water vapor above these mountains was very low. I also had heard a report given by Dr. Gerard Kuiper that the telescopic images of stars were very sharp on Mauna Kea. The substance of the letter was that Jefferies was offering me a full professorship at the University of Hawaii and that he needed answers soon about the design requirements of the telescope.

This was fantastic. This would be an observatory where I believed that the water vapor was perhaps the lowest in the world, except maybe above the mountains in Tibet. The low water vapor meant that the infrared transmission of the atmosphere would be excellent. I jumped at the chance, but first he invited Marge and me to come visit and to see if we would be happy living in Honolulu and if I would enjoy working and teaching in the Physics Department of the University of Hawaii. We went in December and took our son, Alan, who was then less than a year old. We enjoyed the islands and we came back very enthusiastic about the move.

The specifications for the telescope called for it to be 84 inch -0 and +6 inches. Thus, it could be anywhere from 84 inches to 90 inches. It ended up being 88 inches or 2.24 m. Also, it was found that Mauna Kea was much better than Haleakala. Even though access to Mauna Kea was much more difficult, the quality of the astronomical images far outweighed the added difficulty. For the next 24 years, I would spend an average of four nights each month on this mountain. Jefferies arranged to take over a cabin at Hale Pohaku at an elevation of 9,300 feet on the road up the mountain. We would sleep at this lower elevation because it is very difficult to sleep at the top of the mountain due to the lack of oxygen. Working at the top of the mountain was very difficult both mentally and physically. Walking any distance on the mountain top was very tiring. There were stories that circulated about how some astronomers became very confused when working at the top of the mountain. I can tell stories about my own mistakes, but then everyone makes mistakes and anecdotal stories do not give an accurate representation of what astronomers can do at such a superb astronomical site.

It took some time to get the telescope and the building built. We had many problems in getting the telescope running. The building was not completed in time and the telescope had to be stored in a warehouse in Hilo. As a consequence, the plastic wrap that was to protect the paint stuck to the paint and the telescope had to be repainted. When the manufacturers were installing the telescope, the crane slipped and the telescope came crashing down on top of the control room. This scared the wits out of Jim Harwood, who was working inside the room. The tube of the telescope got a big dent in it. The ding had to be banged out much like a dent in a fender, but this steel was 1/8 inch thick. The main gear that drives the telescope was misaligned when it was installed and had to be reground on the mainland. This took a good many months.

The Air Force Cambridge Research Laboratories wanted to have a 24-inch telescope on top of the mountain. So we worked out a deal with them that we would put up a small building for the telescope and maintain it and the telescope in exchange for our using the telescope. They would provide the telescope and would have preemptory use when they needed to use it, which would be only occasionally.

Bob Danielson, an astronomer from Princeton who was spending a sabbatical leave with us, was using the 24-inch for some of his observing. He reported back several things about his physical condition on top of the mountain. First of all, he found that he shouldn't eat a big meal before going up the mountain. Oxygen is required to digest a meal and this requirement puts an additional strain on the heart and lungs. I would find this information to be very useful when I came down with ALS.

It is usual for one to get severe headaches when going up to a high altitude. But Bob found that on succeeding nights after the first night, his headache was much less severe and that he had less malaise. I had noticed this, too, as others had also. I made it a general rule that astronomers should spend a night on the mountain before using a telescope. Jefferies had required us to read a book on high-altitude medicine and physiology. In this book, there was no discussion of an acclimatization occurring within 24 hours. The only acclimatization that was known to occur was an increase in the red blood cells that required two to three months. Yet we found a lessening of headaches and general malaise over 24 to 48 hours. Some years later, after the United Kingdom infrared telescope was built on the mountain, a U.K. physician, Dr. Peter Foerster, tested members of the UK team as they went up and down the mountain. He found a change in the acidity of their urine and he showed that there was an adjustment in their physiology occurring within 24 hours. There was a change in the partial pressure of oxygen in the blood that permitted more oxygen to be assimilated from the air. It is amazing that this acclimatization mechanism had not been discovered with all of the research that was done on high altitude physiology following World War II.

John Jefferies held weekly telescope meetings. They were attended by me, Hans Boesgaard, Walter Bonsack, and other astronomers then on the staff. At one staff meeting, John asked me whether we should have a computer to control the telescope. My immediate reaction was 'no'. One day later, I went back to see him and I told him that after some consideration I was all in favor of computer control. My task then was to draw up specifications for the computer.

I went to the Lincoln Laboratories, which ran a large radio telescope that was controlled by a computer. I wanted to see just how this worked. Actually, the computer didn't immediately run the telescope, but wrote instructions on to a magnetic tape which would control the telescope at a later time. So I was more or less on my own in thinking about just how an operator should operate the telescope through the use of the computer. After getting catalogs from IBM and CDC (a large computer company that is no longer in business), I wrote specifications for all of the computer equipment needed. I asked if we might have a CRT interface (like present-day pc display screens) between the operator and the computer. Only IBM responded to this question and suggested that it it would be about $30,000 for each interface. This was a pretty big chunk of money so we didn't go for that. We added an option to the bid package to quote on testing of the hard drive at a simulated 14,000 foot altitude. They quoted a price of $20,000 for this testing. To their knowledge, hard drives (they were called disk memories in those days) had never been used at such an altitude. The engineers had some serious questions about whether they would work because the read head flies on a film of air over the magnetic coated disk. Sometimes, because of vibration or some disturbance, the head hits the surface of the disk and scrapes up some of the magnetic coating. This is called a crash. It was thought that perhaps the reading head would not fly in the thin air at 14,000 feet. We decided to skip this testing and save $20,000. If the disk didn't work, we could later spend some money for a pressure chamber for it.

One of the tasks that the computer would do was to control the rate that the telescope was driven across the sky. The computer would allow for corrections due to the bending of light by the atmosphere. No telescope drive had ever done that. The computer could also correct for flexure of the telescope structure. A risky task for the computer would be to control the rapid moving of the telescope to the point in the sky where the object is. If something went wrong in this operation, the computer might drive the telescope into the floor of the dome. A relatively simple task for the computer would be the controlling of the rotation of the dome. However, the mathematics of this was not simple as the telescope was not centered in the dome and the the axis of the telescope that pointed parallel to the pole of the earth did not intersect the axis of the telescope that is perpendicular to the direction to the pole. I worked on the trigonometry of this problem off and on for three or four months before hitting upon the solution.

Jim Harwood had worked for the Department of Geophysics on Maui and then on the evaluation of the astronomical quality of the Mauna Kea site. Jefferies suggested that I should consider him as the system software engineer for the 88-inch telescope. This was satisfactory with me as he was very bright. We sent him off to the training school for IBM 1800 program engineers. The IBM 1800, which was very similar to the then popular IBM 1130 that I had used for scientific computing at Lowell, was the computer that we had signed a contract to purchase. By today's standards, it is exceedingly slow. Moreover, it had only 40,000 words of memory. This meant that exchanges between core memory and disk memory were constantly taking place. All this made programming very difficult and subject to many possible errors. That is why it was many years before we would let the computer have control of direct positioning of the telescope. But we did have the computer perform tasks of acquiring the data in between the task of controlling the telescope and the dome. This worked out pretty well. I never wrote a paper on computer control of the telescope which later I regretted.

One afternoon when I returned home from a sojourn on the mountain, Marge told me that my father had died. While I packed, she got me reservations on the 5 p.m. flight from Honolulu to Baltimore. My father was 81. Mom said he died from a heart attack. But it was obvious that he had lost much weight. My mother didn't know why since he wouldn't go to a doctor.

Hawaii is full of vermin. Cockroaches are everywhere. In fact, at a party one night when it was time to leave, I had to walk down the street to my car. The street was illuminated with mercury vapor lights, and the cockroaches were so thick under these lights that it was impossible not to step on them. Our cats were covered with fleas. Every night when I came home from work, I would spend some time combing fleas from our long-haired cat. I would usually get about 50 fleas every evening. We read that there are about 100 times as many fleas in the carpet as are on the cat. Also, there are ground termites and flying termites. Of course, we used many chemicals to control these vermin. So I was exposed to a number of different kinds of pesticides.

I was still very much in the doldrums from having made such a big mistake in the paper about life on Mars. I was very apprehensive about writing further papers. One day, Jefferies called me into his office for a heart-to-heart chat. He told me that my productivity was not up to par. He said that as the Institute grew, I would become unhappy with myself as other productive astronomers joined the staff and would be getting telescope time whereas I would not. I left his office dejected, but I had resigned myself to do something about this. It wasn't long before I got excited about the discovery of volcanoes on Io, a moon of Jupiter. This was through observations by the Voyager spacecraft, but I realized that earlier puzzling infrared measurements were puzzling because of the volcanoes. In fact, I had already written a paper on the puzzling nature.

So during my last 10 years I was fairly productive. I figured out all sorts of ways of observing individual volcanoes even though telescopes were hardly able to see any details on the disk of Io because it is so tiny. I had an undergraduate student and two postdoctoral fellows collaborating with me during this period. I was also fortunate in engaging the collaboration of Charlie Kaminski, a telescope operator at the NASA Infrared Telescope on Mauna Kea. He and I wrote several papers about our infrared observations of Io. Incidentally, Charlie is the very same person who is known as "Choo-choo" Charlie in Jerri Nielson's book "Icebound," which is about her being trapped at the South Pole with breast cancer.

I decided that when I got to age 65, I would retire because I couldn't keep up with the young squirts and after all, they had a right to a job. Being a University of Hawaii professor made me a part of the State employee system and entitled me to their retirement benefits. For every year that I worked for the State, I would get 2 percent of the average of my last three years salary. Moreover, I could purchase additional retirement time for the 2 1/2 years that I spent in the military. That would cost me $9,000, but it was well worth it over the expected time that I would be collecting the pension, so this time was added to the 24 years that I was with the University. I also would get the additional 20% of medical costs beyond the 80% that would be paid by Medicare and I would get 100% percent of the cost of prescriptions except for a small co-payment.

Changes that were made in the tax code about 10 years before my retirement allowed me to buy a tax-sheltered annuity free of tax on the annuity payment part of my salary. For each of these years I bought nearly as much as I was allowed to buy by the tax code. This tax-sheltered annuity was only permitted for teachers and hospital workers. At a later time a change in the tax code allowed me to roll this annuity over into an IRA. I took out my IRA in a mutual-fund.

Not long after Marge and I went to Hawaii we bought a house. After about five years in this house, we sold it and bought another house which was only a few blocks from the University. This, of course, turned out to be a very desirable location. When we sold it 18 years later, its value had increased nine times. The price of housing in Hawaii had been pushed up by the purchases made by Japanese nationals. The Japanese paid whatever the asking price was and did not bargain at all. A friend of mine, who had sold his house, said that the Japanese man who bought it had already bought 30 houses that day. When we sold our house, it was pretty much at the peak of the housing market in Hawaii. Shortly after that, the Japanese realized they had overbought U.S. real estate.

My Aunt Amy had left me a tidy sum in her will. I had invested this in stocks and they had grown in value. All these things left Marge and me a nice nest egg for retirement. I didn't know it then, but this money would come in handy for my ALS.

I've Been Working On The Railroad

(scratch and sniff)

I've been told that a re-encountered smell may evoke the most powerful memory recall. This happened to me in October of 1972 when my family and I visited Griffith Park in Los Angeles and we wound up at the Los Angeles Live Steamers, a group of people who build and run miniature trains that they have constructed to a scale of 1/12 or 1/8 of actual size. What really got to me was the smell of coal smoke and hot lard oil (lubrication for the cylinders) mixed with steam. It brought real locomotives in the train yards in Baltimore back to memory. Never had I seen or smelled model railroads that were so realistic. I knew then and there that I had to build a steam locomotive. I went to a model railroad shop in Pasadena where we were living while I spent a year's sabbatical at the Jet Propulsion Laboratory. I bought a copy of *Live Steam*, a magazine devoted to large scale model railroading. I also saw a partly completed 1/12 scale steam locomotive in their window. It was being sold on consignment by a man who lived in Sierra Madre. I contacted him and bought the engine for $900. It was about half completed. I discovered that there were some problems with the work that had been done on it and I needed to remachine some of the parts. There was still a lot of work to do on it. It took me three years, but I finally completed it. It has about 900 parts, 1000 bolts and nuts, and 1100 rivets.

We were back in Hawaii when I finished it. My yard in Hawaii was very small and also not well suited to putting down a railroad because it was rather sloped. I found that I could get in a 22-foot diameter circle of track, which was about the minimum radius that the locomotive could handle. This would give me some fun nevertheless. My boys and I spent many hours running the train around the circle. A steam engine like this operates at 100 pounds per square inch steam pressure and can pull four or five kids on cars besides the engineer. I built a number of cars; some were flat cars on which I could put seats, one was a gondola car, several were tank cars, and one was a caboose.

When we moved to Flagstaff I made big plans for a railroad. We bought a house on a double lot that was relatively level. It took me a year to put the track down. The track was a loop that was 440 feet around. It went around the house, across the driveway where there was a crossing signal, and even over a trestle. I bought 1,000 feet of appropriate size aluminum rail. Ties were made out of 4 X 4 lumber that I cut lengthwise with a table saw so as to have nine strips of wood from the cross section. These were then cut to into 12 inch lengths, thus yielding 72 ties from each piece of lumber. Altogether the loop of the track has 2200 ties. Before putting the ties down, they were soaked for two weeks in a black preservative solution.

I had a shop built on to the house so that I could have a metal lathe, a drill press, and I planned to get a milling machine. I decided that I would make a new locomotive that would be a model of one of the very first diesel electric locomotives that were made as a joint venture by General Electric, American Locomotive Corp., and Ingersoll-Rand Corp. in 1930. There were plans for a model of this locomotive in a magazine, but I made a number of modifications to the plans so that it was more faithful to the originals. The model locomotive was powered by a storage battery that drove electric motors. I had a hand control at the end of a short cable. I sat on a car that followed the engine and controlled it from there.

This locomotive became my main stay because it was so easy to operate. It didn't require all of the maintenance that the steam locomotive did. I would have to work on the steam locomotive for about an hour after running it, cleaning the flues and cleaning and oiling the moving parts including the inside of the cylinders. It also took 20 or 30 minutes to get steamed up. So I generally ran the new engine. I ran this locomotive about 150 miles. I gave many, many kids rides on the train. It was hard to keep them sitting upright because they tended to lean on the curves. Since the space between the rails, called the gauge, is only 4 3/4 inches, it is very hard to stay on the track unless everyone sits straight up right. It's top speed was three miles per hour for a scale speed of 36 miles per hour, almost identical to the top speed of the original which was 37.

I also took this engine and several cars down to the Maricopa Live Steamers, which had an extensive railroad in McCormick Park in Scottsdale. Their track for my scale train was a 1,100-foot loop. I would run 15 to 20 miles on this track during one of their club meets. They also had track for one-eighth scale which they used to give the public free rides.

Throughout the summer, while I was becoming weaker and weaker from my then unknown disease, I worked on trying to get a spur from my railroad track into my shop. I wanted this so I could store my cars and engine inside and could easily move them outside through a hole in the shop wall. The floor of the shop was above the level of the track and so I had to build a ramp up to the floor level, or actually up to the lowest level of an elevator that would raise a car or an engine up to various levels of a rack which would be inside the shop. The elevator was finished and it worked okay. During the process of building the ramp, Marge helped me mix the concrete and cement the cinder block pillars that would support a bridge to the elevator. Marge also helped me get rocks to build the ramp up to the bridge. I would have to sit on the ground to build what was essentially a rock wall. Marge was a big help in all of this.

But I found that I could not get up from the ground, and I would have to call Marge to come and help me up. Finally, I couldn't do anything more. Sadly, I had to give up my dreams of having the railroad running into the shop. I would have to occupy my time with other things.

In August, I bought a ham radio station that would work on the shortwave bands and allow me to talk to anyone in the world. Using Morse code, I began talking to people everywhere. One of my first contacts was with a ham in Kelsey, Australia. It was fun chewing the rag with people. Typical contacts would include our names, a location, how we are receiving the other station, the weather, sometimes our age, and when we became a ham. Toward the end of the year, I became interested in working DX, that is, foreign countries. But I will tell you more about this in the last chapter.

I Choose To Live

Motor Neuron
and Similar Diseases

Motor neuron diseases affect the motor neurons of the central nervous system. This system includes the brain stem, the upper motor neurons, and the lower motor neurons. The most familiar of these diseases is ALS. There are at least several forms of ALS. One form is of genetic origin and constitutes about 5 to 10% of the ALS cases. This form is called familial ALS or FALS for short. The other kind of ALS is sporadic and is called SALS for short.

There are about 5000 new cases of ALS every year in the U.S. There are about twice as many cases in men as in women. Nobody knows why. Nobody knows why ALS only affects motor neurons. The senses of touch and pain are not impaired. Bladder, bowel, and sexual functions are retained.

There is no definitive test for ALS. The only way of diagnosing ALS is by eliminating all other possible diseases. It usually takes from nine months to a year to make a diagnosis of ALS. If there is no significant treatment or cure for ALS, why care about making an accurate diagnosis? The reason is that there are other diseases that mimic ALS and some of these have effective treatments.

In 1991, a major step forward was made at Northwestern University by researcher Teepu Siddique. He discovered the exact location of the gene on chromosome 22 that is responsible for causing some of the FALS. He later discovered that this gene is responsible for the formation of an enzyme called super oxide dismutase, which is believed to remove free radicals from the body. These free radicals will damage or destroy cells. A defect in the gene causes a defective form of the enzyme to be produced, and it was then thought that the defective form of the enzyme would be ineffective in scavenging for the free radicals. In 1993, Siddique was able to produce a mouse model for ALS, that is, a strain of mice that developed an ALS-like disease. By showing that these mice, when supplied with the correct form of SOD1, as the enzyme is called, still developed ALS. He showed that the defective gene most likely produced an enzyme that was a causative agent. It was then thought that the sporadic form of ALS would have similar causes.

It is known that in SALS there is a build up of glutamate levels in the gaps, called synapses, between motor neurons. Glutamate is the transporter of the nerve message across the gap. After transporting the excitatory message, it is normally removed by glial cells that carry it back to the originating neuron. But if the glutamate remains, it continually excites the following motor neuron. This continued excitation eventually causes the death of the motor neuron. It is interesting to note that the pop, pop, pop that I heard when getting my EMG was the result of the continual excitation of the neuron. A drug, called riluzole, has been developed that regulates the glutamate level. This drug, which is marketed under the name Rilutek, has been shown to slow the progression of the sporadic ALS by about 20%.

There is also an ALS-like disease that occurs on Guam and the Micronesia islands. This has recently been attributed to the consuming of a flour made from the cycad tree. It seems clear to me that there may be many causes for ALS. It is, then, not just one disease but a number of diseases. The defect on chromosome 22 causes only 20 percent of the familial ALS. Another recently discovered gene may be responsible for a few percent of the other FALS. Undoubtedly, causes are varied and complex.

There are other CNS diseases that have similar symptoms to ALS. One of these is spinal muscular atrophy, or SMA, a disease that affects the lower motor neurons. This begins a little earlier in life than ALS, which usually begins between ages 40 and 65. Like ALS, muscle wasting accompanies SMA. The motor neurons nourish the muscle that they connect to. If the neuron ceases to function, then muscle wasting is a consequence.

A disease that affects only the upper motor neurons is primary lateral sclerosis. This usually begins in the 20s or 30s. PLS and SMA do not qualify as ALS because they do not involve both a upper and lower motor neurons. One disease that also mimics some of the ALS symptoms is called the Mattingly disease. In 1640, Thomas Mattingly emigrated from England and settled in Maryland. He brought with him a genetic disease that has afflicted many of the Mattinglys. The disease usually begins at about age 17 and causes progressive paralysis of the legs and arms. However, it does not seem to affect breathing and so is not fatal like most cases of ALS. Although the age of onset is too young to be my disease, I've had my son David, who is interested in genealogy, look for any connections that I may have to the Mattinglys. He could not find any connection. My father's mother died when my father was very young. Her maiden name was Dorr. My son has investigated to see if he could find out whether there was any history of a paralytic disease in her family, but could not find any.

Another disease that is often confused with ALS is multi-focal motor neuropathy. This is an autoimmune disease, that is, the immune system is overactive. In this case, the peripheral motor nerves are attacked and die. Multi-focal motor neuropathies can be treated with drugs that suppress the immune system such as the ones used for organ transplants. Such treatments have been very successful for multi-focal motor neuropathy.

University Medical Center Tucson

It was August 1993. I was sitting in the waiting room on the sixth floor of the University Medical Center in Tucson. Dr. Vengrow had made an appointment for me to see Dr. Lawrence Stern. Marge and I had gotten a temporary patient's card at the first floor lobby. I had checked in at the window and was waiting for my name to be called. Finally, I heard my name and I went up to the nurse who had called it. The nurse led me to a room to take my blood pressure and temperature. She then started asking Marge some questions that should have been addressed to me. But Marge answered them without thinking that the nurse had made an affront to me. I have come to learn that this is a frequent thing. People who are handicapped are often assumed to have lost all of their faculties. We went back out into the waiting room to wait for the call to see the doctor.

I heard "William Sinton" and looked up to see a short middle-aged man in a doctor's coat. I soon learned that Dr. Stern is a kindly, mild-mannered, and compassionate man. His personality is perfectly suited to being a neurologist, a physician who has to deal with patients who often have incurable diseases. Walking slowly with my cane, I followed him back to his examining room, which was at the far end of a corridor of examining rooms. There he introduced me to a visiting colleague from Germany and to a physical therapist who would help with his initial evaluation of me. Marge came along as she had done with most of my visits to the various physicians that I had seen along the way to seeing Dr. Stern.

Dr. Stern took a thorough medical history from me. He asked me if I had twitching anywhere. Yes, I did in my legs. The twitching is called fasciculation. Then he got out of his little hammer and after I crossed my legs he hit me on the knee a number of times. Then, after I had removed my shoe and sock for him, he scratched the sole of my foot with a blunt object. He asked me to stick out my tongue. I later learned that he was looking for twitching of the tongue. Twitching of the tongue would have been indicative of bulbar involvement, which would have been bad. He held a pencil in front of my eyes and asked me to follow it as he moved it to and fro and up and down. He noticed that my eyes unlatched from simultaneous tracking as he moved the pencil. He called to the German doctor to observe the phenomenon of my eyes. He and the German doctor discussed the results of my muscle biopsy and decided that the muscle biopsy didn't tell them anything. Then he said he wanted to get another EMG since the ones I had previously included only one nerve-conduction velocity. He wanted to see more nerve velocities. He called a Dr. Bamford on the phone to set up an appointment for the the EMG, which could not be done until the next day. He wrote out a laboratory requisition for blood tests for Lyme disease, heavy metals, and certain blood enzymes. The physical therapist began testing the strength of my arms by opposing my pushing down and lifting up. She also tested how tightly I could grasp things with my hands.

Dr. Stern confirmed that I had some form of motor neuron disease, but at the time he was not sure which. He wanted to see me again in two months time.

But first, he took me across the hall and introduced me to the managing director of the MDA, the Muscular Dystrophy Association. She said that the Association would loan me a walker. The MDA has ALS as one of the diseases that it looks after. I was now one of "Jerry's Kids."

Next day after the testing, Marge and I went to visit the Sonoran Desert Museum, where we ran into the German doctor again. The Sonoran Desert Museum has many species of desert plants and desert animals and is certainly an interesting place to visit if you are in Tucson.

We went back in November and saw Stern again. Stern came out to greet me again and called out my name. We went back to the same room. I went more slowly now as I was walking with two canes. He introduced me to one of his medical students. A physical therapist was also in the room. She did another evaluation of the strength of my arms and hands. He asked the medical student to tell him what she observed about me. The student was nervous and hesitant, and he had to encourage her in order to get more response. He now asked me to take off a shoe and a sock, and he scratched the sole of my foot again. He asked the student about the Babinski signs and how the location of a lesion in the central nervous system could be found from the motion of the big toe. Again, he asked me to stick out my tongue.

I now questioned him as to whether I had ALS. He said "You have too many symptoms, but tentatively I'll say that you do have an atypical form of ALS." He then gave me a suggestion about taking certain vitamins that were being tested in a program at Harvard to see if they're beneficial for ALS. He said that he would give me a list of them before I left, but apparently this was forgotten, for I did not have the list when I left. When I got back to Flagstaff, my wife called him and he said he would get his secretary to send the list of the vitamins and their dosages. When I received the list, it was typed out on a 8 1/2 by 11 paper, not on a letterhead. There was no identified source of the list of vitamins. I suppose that doctors are not supposed to prescribe vitamins for their patients.

The list included vitamin E, vitamin C, beta carotene, selenium, co-enzyme Q-10, and N-acetylcystiene, all in large amounts. He explained that they were anti-oxidants and that recent work on familial ALS showed that free radicals may have been responsible for causing the death of neurons. It was thought that anti-oxidants, which destroy free radicals, may help to alleviate the effects of ALS.

Marge and I now faced what I think both of us had known was true - I had ALS. We both cried when we spoke of this. But we decided that I still have a life to live and that I was not doing too badly.

One evening, Marge and I were sitting on a bench in an alcove at our front door. In this alcove, we had some mementos such as a tiki, a large piece of petrified wood, and a volcanic bomb. A volcanic bomb is a piece of lava that has been thrown from a volcano and shaped by its motion through the air while still in a semifluid state. I had found this piece of lava near the top of Mauna Kea. For many years, it sat in the front yard of our home in Honolulu. I brought it along when I moved back to Flagstaff. According to Hawaiian legend, this is a no-no. In the Visitor's Center of the Volcanoes National Park on the Big island of Hawaii, they have an exhibit of items that were returned to the Park Rangers and which originally came from one of the volcanoes. Each of the items was accompanied by a letter that stated what terrible hard luck that the thief had had. This legend was known as the curse of Madame Pele who is the goddess of the volcanoes.

It suddenly became obvious to me that this volcanic bomb might be the source of all my troubles. I am a scientist of course, but I am going to play all of the percentages. I told Marge what I was thinking. The next day I called the superintendent of the Mauna Kea Observatory and asked him if he could find a home for the bomb. He said he would and Marge packed up the bomb and sent it off to him. It now resides in the visitor's area of the 2.2-m University of Hawaii telescope. However, my ALS still progresses.

At a previous session, Stern had suggested that I read books by Dr. Bernie Siegel, which I had done already. One of the things that Siegel says in his books is that if the placebo effect is real, which it is, then why not use it. It doesn't matter whether drugs are proven effective by double-blind studies, if they work, they work. Stern had convinced me of the effectiveness of the high dosage vitamins. When I returned to Flagstaff and began taking the vitamins, I began looking for signs of improvement, but after some weeks I decided that I was still getting weaker.

Dr. Stern had also written a prescription for a foot support to compensate for my foot drop. I took it to an orthopedic shop in Flagstaff. They gave me a temporary off-the-shelf set of AFOs which stands for ankle foot orthodics. They also made casts for custom-made AFOs that would have metal springs. When I got them three weeks later, I was much weaker and they were so heavy that I could not use them. They billed Medicare for $1,000 apiece for them, but Medicare cut the cost to $700 for each.

In October, 1992, when I was beginning to have trouble walking, I was looking for a way to get exercise. Marge got us a family membership in the Flagstaff Athletic Club and I began swimming there. I would swim in their pool for 20 or 30 minutes. I could do this without putting much stress on my feet and the foot drop didn't bother me. I would swim two or three times a week. It was very invigorating and I could get my heart rate up to the aerobic level. After swimming in the pool, I would go to the Jacuzzi and spend about 10 minutes in the hot water.

When I started anti-oxidant vitamins, I began to notice that I was getting a rash after swimming. I discovered that they were putting bromine in the water instead of chlorine. I remembered from my chemistry courses and from my other readings on chemistry that bromine was a very corrosive chemical on the skin. If liquid bromine was put on the skin, even vigorous washing would not remove all of it. The chemicals that are added to the swimming pool and to the Jacuzzi water produce some free bromine in the water. It seemed stupid to me to be taking anti-oxidants while sitting in the pool of a very strong oxidizing agent such as bromine.

In mid-December, I found that it was almost impossible to get out of the swimming pool even by pulling myself up on the railing alongside the stairs that led into the pool. The last time I went swimming I had to get somebody to pull me out of the pool. I decided that I had better give up swimming as I didn't know whether I might drown.

By this time, I also needed a walker. Sometimes, I would use the two canes because it was faster, but mostly

I used the walker. But on Christmas Eve, 1993, I fell down twice with a walker. I knew then that I would have to give up using the walker. My wife rented a wheelchair for me. Ever since then, I have been in a wheelchair.

When I saw Dr. Stern in February, I was, of course, in the rented wheelchair. This time he didn't call out my name but came directly to me. Again we went to his back room where he had a medical student whom he questioned about my condition.

Although Dr. Stern could not do anything that would help my condition medically, every time I went to him I seemed to be uplifted spiritually. He wanted me to come back every three or four months. I don't think I went back until the following fall. The occasion was a lecture for the MDA about new treatments for various nervous and muscular disorders. Dr. Stern and one of his students would be speaking. The student discussed the recent discovery of prions, which are very small bits of protein that can reproduce themselves. They represent a new form of disease agent and they are believed to cause several diseases, scrapies in sheep, mad cow disease, and Creuzfeldt-Jakob disease in humans. These bits of protein are very indestructible, even boiling will not destroy them. Only incineration will destroy them. New science like this always interests me.

The previous afternoon I had seen Dr. Stern and he had a student with him. The student was a student in neurology so the questions were more detailed. When I stuck out my tongue this time, they discussed it in some detail, but they concluded that it was not twitching. By now, my big toe would not move at all so the Babinski test was meaningless.

When I saw Stern in the spring of 1995, Rilutek, the first drug that was shown to be effective in treating ALS, was being released for early access. I asked him to get me on the list for this drug. I began taking Rilutek in October, 1995. This drug was only expected to increase the lifespan by two or three months, but it seemed worth it. Early Access, the government subsidized program for Rilutek, ended in January, 1996. I had to pay for it or get my insurance to cover it. It was not on my insurance company's list of drugs that they would cover. In a couple of months, Rilutek was added to the list, and since then I have been able to get a three-month supply for $15 copayment. Otherwise, the cost would be about $700 for a month's supply.

The evaluation of Rilutek counted the percentage of patients that had not reached the end point in the nine-month testing period. The end point was considered to be when the patient died or the patient had to be put on a ventilator. I have been on a ventilator for over three years. So I would have been considered the same as being dead. The results of an 18-month test showed that the drug extended the time to the end point by 30 percent. I don't really know how much good Rilutek is doing, but my disease is progressing very slowly.

There have been other drugs that have been tested. Myotrophin is one that initially showed promise. But after questionable results, the FDA refused to approve it for general release. The company, Cephalon, discontinued production of it and left many users, who had been on Early Access, stranded.

On one my trips to see Dr. Stern, he suggested that I should have a pulmonologist so that there would be an evaluation of my vital capacity before it began to decline. That left me very depressed because I had assumed that I might escape problems with breathing. Stern doesn't always cheer me up.

I Choose To Live

Terror in the Home

"I've learned:

That life is tough, but I'm tougher."

Andy Rooney

We didn't want to continue to have to rent a wheelchair. We went to our favorite medical supplier. He suggested that I could get Medicare to pay for the wheelchair, but I would have to get a doctor's prescription. Marge and I called upon my primary care physician for the prescription and he sent us to the hospital rehab center. Here, I saw an occupational therapist, Denise, and a physical therapist, Melissa, who measured me for the wheelchair. It would seem that a manual wheelchair would be an off-the-shelf item, so to speak. But no, it took six weeks to get the wheelchair. It was fortunate that we had rented the wheelchair by the month. Denise and Melissa suggested that we could get Home Health Care to help us. We found that we could get a certified nurse's aide to come in for two hours several times a week. So we called and they agreed to come help us.

The following Monday morning a nurse came to the door to checkup on my condition. She took my blood pressure, my temperature, my pulse, and measured my oxygen concentration with a device called an oximeter. She had no sooner left then the CNA came. I had never had a CNA come visit me before. Since she was going to give me a shower she told me that she was going to see me naked. I suppose she thought that the shock would help me get over my embarrassment.

While this was going on Klaus, another nurse, came to the door. Apparently, his role was to check up on the CNA and on the previous nurse. Finally the CNA, whose name was Madeleine, took me back and gave me a shower. Marge had bought me a shower chair that had wheels and doubled as a commode. She had also gotten a long ramp that led up to the shower stall to a wooden floor that a handyman had made for us. The wooden floor was at the level of the 3 inch high lip underneath the shower door. Madeleine did see me naked and gave me a good shower, even though I found I was getting weak at the end of it.

Since I was unable to stand, she moved me to my bed to get my clothes back on. She had a curious way of pulling my pants up over my hips. She pulled the pants up as for as she could. Then she placed her hands on either side of my hips and pushed down hard on the mattress. She suddenly released her hands and grabbed the waist of my pants and pulled them up as my hips bounced up in the air.

Then an occupational therapist came. She was interested in my radio equipment and how I could work it and whether I needed any assistive devices for that. She also went out into my shop and I showed her my lathe. I showed her how I had been building railroad equipment. I thought I could still operate my lathe, but, in fact, I never used my lathe again.

The last visitor from home health was the physical therapist, Louise, who was a redhead. She wanted to work on the range of motion of my legs. We moved back to my bed again. She picked up one of my legs holding the knee so it would remain stiff. As she raised it, I screamed. My muscles had gotten very tight. She raised it and placed my foot on her shoulder. All the while I screamed. With my foot still on her shoulder, she proceeded to pull the front of my foot up, stretching the muscles in my calf. I screamed even louder. She put my leg back down and pulled up my knee making a vee of my leg. Then she pushed my knee across the other knee thus twisting my spine. Actually, this felt tension relieving and was a welcome change. But soon she was back to raising my leg again and bending my foot. More screaming, but she managed to get my leg a little higher. Then, the horrible process was repeated with the other leg. This ended the parade into our house for that day.

Later on I learned that everyone who knew Louise as a PT referred to her as the "Terror." However, her main purpose was to teach Marge how to do the exercises on me. She came back several more times. Marge began doing these leg exercises three times each week.

I told Louise that repetitious exercise of my muscles seemed to weaken them permanently. Recently, I received a paper from Harry Gould, a PALS of Mesa, Arizona. Harry presented an interesting idea. He supposed that when one exercises, one builds up more glutamate molecules in the synapses and this leads to further destruction of the neurons. This would explain the fact that I seem to get weaker after exercising and that I never recovered my strength. This view of the weakening effect of exercise is certainly not the view of many in the medical profession. Dr. Hiroshi Mitsumoto, a specialist in the care of ALS patients, has stressed the need for exercise. But most of the PALS that I have talked to have said that repetitious exercise causes them to get weaker.

I explained my impression that I lost strength after exercising to Louise. This didn't seem to sink in because at a later time she brought a bicycle device that would fasten to the front of my wheelchair. I told her that I positively would not use this because such an exercise would weaken me further.

Medicare was paying for the home health aide. The nurse would come weekly to checkup on my health. She told us that they would only allow eight weeks for the CNA to come because I was not in critical need of their service. Also, they told me that I couldn't go out except to visit a doctor. I didn't give much attention to this poor advice.

My caregivers now regularly give me range of motion exercises. I am quite limber. I can't imagine what I would look like if I had not kept up with these exercises. I would probably be all twisted up from contraction of muscles. By and large, when the caregivers move my legs and arms, I have only the good feeling of muscles being stretched and without much pain.

Multi Focal
Motor Neuropathy

Sometimes it is not possible to put things together in a chronological fashion when they occur simultaneously. This is the case of the story in this chapter and the stories in the next two chapters. They all happened at about the same time.

I made a trip to see the wise old Dr. Stern in the fall of 1996. He discussed with me again the importance of getting the right diagnosis. He was still not happy with the diagnosis of ALS because I was doing so well at still being alive. He sent me off to get another EMG. I was unable to get this done until the next day. Again, I was stuck with needles and given electric shocks. About 20 inches were marked off along one arm and electrodes placed at the bottom of that. The shock was administered at the upper end of the marks on my arm. The computer showed how fast the impulse traveled down my arm. He gave me shocks all over the place. One that he gave me on my neck was particularly painful, but he had warned me that it would be.

He had an East Indian student with him. They were discussing the results and the student said out loud that I didn't have ALS. We asked the doctor about this and he said he thought I had a treatable disease.

We couldn't see Dr. Stern anymore that week so we returned to Flagstaff. We found out everything we could about multi-focal motor neuropathy on the Internet. This disease was one suggested by the physical medicine physician that gave me the EMG. We found out that it was an auto immune disease, a disease in which the body's own defenses recognize a part of the body as foreign. We found out that the treatment for multi-focal motor neuropathy uses the same drug that is given transplant patients in order to prevent them from rejecting the new organ. We called Dr. Stern and he gave me a prescription for azathioprine. I began taking this and also having, my CBC (red and white blood cells) monitored, which is a precautionary measure.

The real test for whether one has multi-focal motor neuropathy or not is whether the the immune-suppressant drug works or not. Marge and I were elated with the good news and we told everybody. We waited expectantly for something to happen - for me to be able to move my hands again - but this never happened. I went to see Dr. Stern again in about three months and though he was willing to extend the prescription for another three months, he knew that it was not working. In another two months, I knew that too.

Bottoms Up

"Humpty Dumpty sat on a wall

Humpty Dumpty had a big fall

All the king's horses and all the king's men

Couldn't put Humpty Dumpty together again."

Nursery rhyme

We all do dumb things. They are very embarrassing at the time, but later on these pratfalls become the sources of humorous stories. In this chapter, I tell several stories of accidents that happened to me.

While I was still walking around with one cane I went out front to get the mail out of the mailbox and while there I dropped my cane. I bent down to pick up the cane and continued right on down to the ground. I lay there for a bit pondering what to do. Eventually, I decided I would crawl over to a nearby rock that would act as a low seat. I did this, remembering to bring my cane along. I was able to crawl up on to rock and then with my cane I could get myself to a standing position.

Once, when I was in my two-cane mode, I was downtown and I heard a friend's voice calling to me from behind. I turned around from the hips, and to my surprise, I continued right on down to the ground like a corkscrew. It had not occurred to me that I didn't have enough strength to overcome the twisting motion. How embarrassing!

The worst fall I ever had was on of the concrete floor in our garage. One of the previous owners of our house had kept the garage floor waxed and it was somewhat slippery. One day Marge and I were cleaning up things in the garage, and I believe it was at the time that I was using a cane that had a metal tip. This was a poor choice for use on a waxed concrete floor. Well, the cane slipped out and I went head long to the floor. I fell straight forward stiff legged and couldn't get my hands in place to break my fall. My forehead hit the concrete with a thud! Marge was scared out of her wits, but fortunately I didn't lose consciousness. After about 30 seconds, I got myself around to a sitting position and surveyed my damage. I was beginning to get a welt on my forehead and it was skinned, and my nose was bleeding badly. I asked Marge to get me a towel and some ice cubes. I wrapped the towel around the ice cubes and held it against my nose, which soon stopped the bleeding. I really was not too badly hurt. For the rest of the day, I was looking for signs of a concussion, but I didn't seem to get a concussion.

When I was still in my manual wheelchair, Marge got a lift seat for me. This consisted of two boards with a hinge between them. There was a spring arrangement such that when the boards were placed in a chair and one sat on them, the spring would be compressed. When the person got up, the spring would help push him to a standing position. Well, once when I was in the wheelchair with this spring seat under me, I leaned forward to pick up something and thereby took most of my weight off the spring seat which pushed me forward. The next thing I knew I had fallen on to my head.

After I got my powered wheelchair, I was measured for arm supports which would hold my arms up so that I could work with my hands. I would be able to lift things to my mouth and move my hands inward and outward from my chest. It was a spindly contraption with weights and counterbalances and had troughs that my forearms were strapped into. Melissa, the PT, measured the strength of the muscles in my arms, up-down and side-to-side, to see if I would be able to work it when I got the one that was tailored for me. Two or three months later Melissa brought the new arm supports. She affixed the supports to the back of my chair and then adjusted them to fit me. By that time I had become a bit weaker. I couldn't seem to get the hang of using them. My arm would suddenly shoot outward and then, as I tried to bring it back, it would shoot into my chest. Melissa suggested that I practice with it and then I would become proficient with it.

So I tried using it. I could do maybe a few things with it. Then one evening, I tried using it to eat dinner. I could handle my fork with difficulty. Then I tried to pick up my coffee mug. As I brought it unsteadily toward my lips, my hand rotated and the mug turned upside down and spilled the coffee down my front. There had been no measurements of the twisting force that my arms could exert and probably my rotator muscles had become weaker. So the devices ended up in the closet with all the other assistive devices. Every handicapped person has a closet full of gadgets that did not work for them. About one-third of assistive devices fall into this category.

Some months earlier, when I had been using the manual wheelchair, Marge would settle me back into my chair by tilting it all way back until the handles were on the floor. One night, when it was almost time for me to check into one of the ham radio nets, she did this and was unable to get me back upright again. The net began to start, and I needed to make an announcement at the beginning of the net. Marge got me the handy-talky, and while lying with my back on the floor and my feet up in the air, I used the handy-talky to make the announcement.

After the net was over, Marge used the Hoyer lift to pick me up and put me back into my chair. The lift consists a hydraulic cylinder which extends between an overhead arm that connects to a sling and a U shaped frame that is on wheels and will slide under a bed or around a wheelchair. The Hoyer lift is one of the best investments we ever made.

Speaking of assistive devices, a very useful device is the Beezey Board. This consists of a round seat that will rotate and slide along the board. These are called transfer boards, but most transfer boards consist simply of a hardwood board with no moving parts. The object of a transfer board is to allow transfer from a bed to a chair. One virtue of the Beezey Board is that the seat slides very easily because it is made of Teflon.

Once, Marge was spending three days with her sister in Cleveland and I had several nurses to look after me while she was gone. One nurse thought she knew better than I how to do things. We had already had several run-ins. Now, when she was putting me to bed one evening, I was halfway along the Beezey Board. In other words, I was between the chair and the bed. She started to take the chair away. I said, "If you do that, I will be on the floor." She said, "Oh no," and pulled away the chair. I was on the floor. I tried to tell her about getting the Hoyer, but she would have nothing to do with a device that she had not used before. So she went outside and across the street and got a neighbor to come in and help pick me up off the floor.

It was around Christmas and I had only been in my powered wheelchair for a short time. The boys and Marge had gone out to do some shopping while I stayed at home. Well, I managed to run down the Christmas tree. I was buried in it and my hand had been pushed away from the control so I could not back away. I leaned forward with my head and grabbed my sleeve with my teeth to pull my hand up, but then I couldn't get my head back up. So I stayed there for about an hour and a half until the family came home. That was a miserable experience. I thought they would never get home.

I believe that everyone who gets a powered wheelchair has a problem controlling it at first. We ended up getting metal guards put on all the door jambs. Sometimes wheelchairs seem to have a mind of their own. I call my present one Chuckie after the devilish character in the movie. A PALS friend of mine couldn't get the hang of her wheelchair either. She called it Darth.

At another time, I was moving up to the dining-room table and the chair got away from me. I ran into the table and the table hit the control lever such that I couldn't pull it back. The chair pushed the table and all six dining chairs over against the wall. It broke off table legs and accordioned much of the rest of the table. When Marge came home, I met her on the way in and told her, "I have a good news and bad news. The good news is that I'm OK; the bad news is that the dining-room table is not."

My most embarrassing pratfall happened while I was on the toilet. I leaned forward, I suppose in an effort to exert some force that my weak stomach muscles couldn't. I fell forward on to my head and wedged myself between the toilet and shower stall. I called to my wife who came and saw my predicament. We didn't think that she could pick me up without some danger to my neck, which was supporting much of my weight. So I asked her to call 911. She called them but asked them not to use their sirens as it was not that much of an emergency. Well, they did use their sirens, and I guess that always happens if you call 911. A fire engine came and an ambulance came. Suddenly, our bathroom was as populated as Times Square. My butt, of course, was up in the air. Marge had placed a towel over it.

With a person on either side of me, they managed to get me back up on the toilet. And then one of the EMTs gave me a lecture about getting a strap to hold me from falling forward while on the toilet.

Breathing, Swallowing, High Blood Sugar, and Edema

"I've learned:

That life is like a roll of toilet paper. The closer it gets to the end, the faster it goes."

Andy Rooney

After Dr. Stern advised me that I should contact someone about my breathing, I made an appointment with Dr. Joseph Colorafi, one of two pulmonologists in Flagstaff. Dr. Colorafi had me go to the laboratory at the hospital where he and a respiratory technician made a variety of tests of my breathing. The technician took a sample of my arterial blood for a blood gas analysis. This sample is obtained by sticking the needle into the artery at the wrist. The artery is not easy to find and the searching for it is usually accompanied by some pain. The result of the blood gas analysis was that I had a decreased oxygen amount and a normal carbon dioxide amount in my blood. In a way, this was good news because often a PALS will have a normal oxygen amount and an increased carbon dioxide level, which means that the PALS has adapted to decreased breathing.

The breathing tests showed that I had a normal sucking ability, but I only had about 60% of my vital capacity, which is the total amount of air I can breathe in. Dr. Colorafi requested that I come back three months later

99

to repeat the tests to see what the changes were. They were pretty much the same and so he had me make an appointment to see him in his office in about three months.

He had Stephanie, a respiratory therapist, in his office when I arrived there. Stephanie made a measurement of my vital capacity. This entailed my sucking and blowing through a contraption that was connected to a computer. She put this thing in my mouth and said suck, suck, suck, keep sucking, keep sucking, now blow, blow, blow, keep blowing, keep blowing, and OK stop. The computer printed out a graph of my sucking and blowing and showed that my vital capacity was about 60%. A. normal person has a vital capacity of about 85% on this test.

Dr. Colorafi reviewed the findings with me and then suggested that I should go on a Bipap respirator at night time. This machine keeps a positive pressure on the lungs, even during expiration. This keeps the lungs inflated at all times. Stephanie brought this equipment to our house and explained its workings. The device was connected by a hose to a well-fitting mask that went over my nose. I didn't use the Bipap during the daytime because it was impossible to talk with it on.

We had problems with it at night because I couldn't keep my mouth shut, and much of the air pumped by the Bipap escaped through my mouth. We tried putting a stout rubber band over the top of my head and underneath my chin, but still my mouth would fall open. This was when I was sleeping on my back, but several hours during the night I would sleep on my side and then I didn't keep the Bipap on because of pressure on my nose. By this time, I would have to wake Marge to turn me over so I would have her change the Bipap at that time. I went on this way for several months.

In April, 1997, we planned a trip to Sacramento California with a stopover in Death Valley on the way. We were about to leave on this trip, but I was showing signs of not being able to breathe well. First, Marge arranged to have oxygen bottles for our trip. But on the weekend before we were to leave, I seemed to be having a lot of trouble breathing and Marge and I went off to the hospital emergency room. They took X-rays of my chest and they thought I had fluid in my right lung. A respiratory therapist came in and began thumping on the side of my chest to break the fluid loose. While this was going on, someone was trying to insert an IV in my arm, and someone else was fitting a Bipap to my face. When someone else came along with yet another task to do at same time, I told them to quit. This was a scene straight out of "ER."

A number of nurses tried to get the IV in but to no avail. They gave up and a decision was made to admit me and move me over to the respiratory ICU. More X-rays were taken and Dr. Colorafi, who had been called, planned to go in with a cystoscope and suction out the fluid. He also suggested to me that I should consider getting a tracheostomy, which we had discussed previously in his office. A tracheostomy is a hole into the trachea (windpipe) at the base of the neck. He discussed this again and said that even if they fixed my present problems, I would be back there again in a few months. Before Colorafi left the hospital, I had opted for the tracheostomy. I wanted to live all the more now because my grandchild would be born to David and Missy in a few weeks. They had opted not to know whether it would be a boy or girl until birth. Nevertheless they already had a name: Aaron or Erin.

I had gone to the ER on Saturday. At this point, I stopped taking the immunosuppressant. It was not doing me any good anyhow. The tracheotomy (the operation to create a tracheostomy) was performed on Monday by Dr. Jerry Mohr. When I came to, I was connected to this hideous machine, a ventilator that was made for all purposes. It seemed to be banging and thumping and the hose that went to my throat was jumping up and down with every breath. Marge showed up almost as soon as I woke up. A nurse came, and since I was having difficulty breathing, she suctioned secretions and some blood out of my windpipe. She told me that suctioning was irritating to the windpipe and should not be done too often. But she didn't have to tell me about being irritated because I already knew that.

Dr. Colorafi came to visit me. He wanted me to breathe on my own for 20 minutes. This was a strain on me, though I managed to do it. He told me that I didn't have fluid in my lung, but that my right lung was partially collapsed. They got it re-expanded.

That afternoon, a speech therapist, Kim Allen, came to visit me. She was overjoyed when she found out that they had put in a fenestrated cannula. This is a curved piece of plastic tubing that goes through the hole in my throat and curves downwards toward my lungs. A fenestrated cannula has a window midway along its length to let air pass through toward the vocal cords. This cannula, when combined with a valve called the Passy-Muir valve, would allow me to speak in whole sentences. Kim had brought such a valve to give me. Since I wouldn't be talking for a while because of a swollen throat, she brought some things that had text that I might point to to make my needs known. Earlier, one of my ALS friends, who was on a ventilator, showed me that he could make a clucking sound with his mouth to get someone's attention. I remembered this and put it to good use. One night, I had a terrible time getting the nurse's attention to suction me. I couldn't use the call button because I couldn't move my hands. I finally got a cardiopulmonary technician who came to check on me.

The cannula that I spoke of above is called the outer cannula, and it stays in my throat for about three months before it is changed for a new one. Surrounding the outer cannula at its interior end is a doughnut-shaped balloon. A tiny tube is connected to the balloon and this comes outside to a connection to which a syringe can be connected. The balloon can be inflated to block around the end of the cannula and prevent air moving beyond the end of the cannula. An inner cannula is generally inserted through the outer cannula. It can be either fenestrated or solid. With a solid cannula and with the balloon inflated, the air path from the lungs through the mouth is completely cut off. An air path through the solid cannula does exist. The ventilator is connected to this.

In the late afternoon after surgery, the ICU nurse came in to put a feeding tube down through my nose and into my stomach. They tried one nostril, but it got stuck and so they finally got it through the other nostril. They had to take an X-ray to see whether the end of the tube really was in my stomach. However, a radiologist had to read the X-ray and this took hours because she was off to dinner. So finally I could eat. I had an appetizing meal of stuff shoved down the tube. My throat would have to heal a lot more before I could chew solid food.

In a day or two, they let me eat a puree of foods. To each item on the plate, they added a very strong dark blue dye. The purpose of the dye was to find out if any of the food leaked through my epiglottis (that's the little valve in the throat that cuts off the path to the windpipe when one swallows). They would find out if this valve leaked if any of the blue dye showed up when they suctioned me. I had a number of meals this way.

They wanted to get me up into my wheelchair. Marge had brought the Hoyer to the hospital. She picked me up from my bed and put me into my chair and I stayed there for about an hour. Of course, I had on a hospital gown which was open in the back. I hadn't had a bowel movement since I was put into the hospital. When they picked me up, I couldn't help myself and pooped on the floor. The poop was green because of all the blue dye. The nurse called in the hospital cleaning staff and they took a look at this and walked away. It became something of a cause for the cleaning people who didn't want to clean up the mess.

Since Marge was going to be my principal caregiver, they taught her everything about suctioning. First of all there are two kinds of catheters, the in-line catheter and the removable catheter. The in-line catheter has a T at the throat. The air comes in from one side. Directly opposite the throat, is a soft plastic tubing, about 1 inch diameter, with a catheter running through the middle and sealed to the outer plastic hose at the lower end. To suction, one pushes the inner catheter tubing down the throat collapsing and accordioning the outer tubing. The catheter tubing is connected to a suction machine and the secretions in the windpipe are suctioned out. Breathing is cut off from the time that the suction tube is inserted until the time that it is removed, about 15 seconds later.

The removable catheter is inserted through the inner cannula and pushed down into the windpipe. The disadvantage of this is that the connection to the breathing hose has to be broken and more time is required to make a suctioning. The advantage of the removable catheter is that it is much easier to maintain.

The in-line catheter is preferred because of exposure to diseases which occur in the hospital environment. In the home environment, this exposure doesn't exist and only exposures to every day dust, pollen, germs, and viruses, to which our bodies already have some immunity, occur. In the home environment, it is only necessary to keep catheters clean. While sterility is attempted, it is recognized that such a goal is very difficult to achieve. But after all, we all are exposed to these sources of infection.

They swapped a Respironics SLV-102 ventilator for the noisy ventilator that had been supplying the breathing for me. This was the unit that I would be taking home. It would be rented from Respironics and paid for by Medicare. This is the same ventilator used by Christopher Reeve and was often shown in the movie "Rear Window."

Stephanie, the respiratory therapist, wanted Marge to use the in-line catheter because she believed it would be simpler. So for about two weeks after I got home, we used the in-line catheter. We changed to external catheters because they were softer and not so hard on my windpipe.

After more than a week in ICU, I got to go home. It was very difficult at first with all the cleaning of tubing, catheters, and cannulas. It took me about two weeks or more to get used to suctioning, which has to be done about a dozen times each day. By using the solid cannula at night with the balloon inflated, I can sleep through the night without needing suctioning. If I do need suctioning in the middle of the night, I make my clucking sound which awakens Marge.

Aaron was born about three weeks after I got out of the hospital. He was so tiny even though it was several weeks later before I saw him. One of the first trips I made with the ventilator was to see Aaron. David and Missy live in Kanab, Utah, only 200 miles away.

Now for a dog story. I have two dogs. One is a golden retriever, which we got as a pup about four years ago. Her name is Cicely after Cicely, the fictitious town in "Northern Exposure." Our other dog, Tucsie, is a collie mix that we inherited from a neighbor. We began teaching Cicely tricks while she was still a puppy. She learned very well. Sometimes after Marge has gotten me into bed and she goes to a far part of the house to put laundry into the washing machine, occasionally I will need suctioning. During this period, I make my clucking sound but Marge doesn't hear me. After I do this a second time, Cicely will get off of Marge's bed and Tucsie will come out from under my bed and both will run into the laundry room to get Marge. We did not teach the dogs to do this. Apparently, they realized that I needed help from someone else, and so they go running for Marge. On some occasions, when Marge is away and a caregiver is looking after me, the dogs will wake up the caregiver. One very fortunate thing is that I can breathe on my own for quite some time. Therefore, it is not necessary to make a quick suctioning. I have plenty of time for making transfers when going to bed, without needing to maintain my connection to the ventilator.

It has been more than three years since I had the tracheotomy operation. Immediately after the operation, I was feeling better than I had felt in the previous year. With more air in my lungs, I was digesting my food better. And, of course, I had more energy.

I am very lucky not to have the bulbar onset form of the ALS. I am not sure what my outlook would be if I had that, but I guess with my spirit, I would be doing pretty well. My swallowing is still fair, but I do have some trouble occasionally with pills becoming stuck in my throat. I have found that V-8 juice is the best drink for swallowing pills. If the pill does get stuck, I chew up some string cheese and that seems the best thing to get stuck pills down. I have to chew my food very finely before swallowing or I am apt to choke. If I get too much in my mouth, I'm apt to get some up my nose. This occurs because the Passy-Muir valve forces my breath out of my nose and mouth. If food is in the way it goes up my nose. I've had corn kernels come out of my nostrils.

Several years ago I noticed that after eating sweet foods, my heart began racing and I felt a shortness of breath, especially if I did not have oxygen. I realized that sugary foods put a sudden demand for oxygen to metabolize them. I remembered back to the nights on Mauna Kea and the story about not eating heavy meals before going up the mountain. I didn't know that the shortness of breath problem went further than not having sufficient oxygen. Later on, I read in the ALS Digest that PALS have a tendency toward glucose intolerance. This is sort of like diabetes but the pancreas is not involved. The theory is that since ALS patients have lost muscle mass they have also lost insulin receptors that are attached to the muscle. Thus there is decreased ability to store insulin.

Marge and I talked to my primary care physician about this, and he suggested that we buy a glucometer and measure my glucose levels. It turned out that they were running moderately high (240) an hour-and-a-half after a meal. The normal range is 80 to 140, so this was too high. I now take quick-acting insulin with each meal and this has cut the glucose level. This has also made a great improvement in my well being.

It seemed that as soon as I began having trouble walking, my feet began to swell. In fact, they were swelling despite my taking daily walks. I've wondered whether the swelling was the source of my decreased motor control. Anyhow, the edema became rather severe in my upper and lower limbs. I developed a small pressure sore on one my toes and it became deeper and wouldn't heal. It was infected with an unusual bacteria which they treated by giving me Cipro and Clindamycin. The redness went away, but the sore healed very slowly. What made a big difference in the healing was restoring circulation in my legs. The circulation had been compromised by the edema. Dr. Wiebe, my podiatrist, sent me to a lymphedema clinic to reduce my edema. So I now have my leg wrapped every day. This has reduced the swelling and I can even see veins. My sore is almost gone.

Pressure sores, commonly called bedsores, are generally very difficult to treat. It is fortunate that PALS do not lose their sense of feeling and can either move themselves if they begin to hurt or get someone to shift their position. I have a marvelous cushion for my chair and an air mattress for my bed. I rarely need shifting with these super soft things under me.

Getting Out And Traveling

Nine O'clock Coffee

Poem about the coffee group

at the Weatherford Hotel

by Robert Senseman

At exactly 9:30 a.m., Henry takes a spoon and raps it against a bowl to get everyone's attention, and we play the game. Henry, who is in his 90's and is a retired astronomer from Lowell Observatory, has taken out his watch that has been set in accordance with time signals from the National Bureau of Standards station WWV.

Every Tuesday morning at 9:00 a.m., you may find me with a bunch of cronies at the Weatherford Hotel. I have a white Dodge Caravan that has been outfitted by IMS (Independent Mobility Systems of Farmington, NM) for handicapped people. It kneels. I call it "Squat." A pneumatic system allows the rear suspension to collapse. With the van's lowered floor, the ramp has only to rise about five inches to allow my wheelchair to roll in. My caregiver takes me downtown to the hotel and leaves me there while I join my buddies. Most of them are up in years.

The purpose of the game is to determine who will pay for coffee. The game is run by the person who paid for the coffee on the previous day. It is a number a game. The number, which has been chosen by the person running the game, is between 1 and 1000. The number has been written on the underside of a paper napkin so that only the person running the game knows the number. The game runs around the table generally starting to the left of the game runner. The first person chooses a number in the range 1-1000. The game runner says whether the number is higher or lower than the correct number. The next person has to choose within the narrowed range that includes the number. And again, the game runner tells whether it is high or low. It doesn't take long to narrow the range so that someone is forced to pick the correct number. The game generally runs through about 10 to 15 people. The one who wins the game has the honor to pay for the coffee. Surprisingly, it can be a lot of fun. Also, it's only rarely that I have to pay for coffee.

Marge and I generally go out to eat about once a week. I think that one of the real pleasures in life is eating. It really makes life worth living. I enjoy seafood, all except for shrimp, which I like but to which I am allergic. Fortunately, we have a few good restaurants in Flagstaff. There are some good steak houses and sometimes we get good fish and other seafood.

Those of us that have severe physical handicaps still have a brain. It is the human brain that distinguishes us from other animals. The familiar phrase "A brain is a terrible thing to waste," is certainly true. I believe the brain needs nourishment from the senses. We need handshakes, hugs, kisses, smells (both good and bad), the taste of food, beauty, reading, music, a babbling brook, hearing poetry and many other things that make our life enjoyable.

I believe that the communication between humans produces a greater being than is possible with the isolated brain. My higher being is the collective power of all of humanity. If the brain is not stimulated, it becomes reclusive, paranoid, and doesn't contribute to society. I think that it is imperative that handicapped people get out and remain part of the society.

This is the 10th anniversary of the American Disabilities Act. There have been notable improvements in accessibility to establishments in Flagstaff. A major reconstruction of the sidewalks in the downtown area has provided for ramp access at street corners. But some restaurants and shops that I would like to go to are simply not accessible to me. They were built before the American Disabilities Act came into effect.

I believe that there has been some backlash effect of the Act. It seems to me that there is only partial compliance with the law in some shopping malls. Marge and I went out to a grocery store at a shopping mall. We parked in a handicapped parking stall next to a yellow crosshatched walkway. My wife had pulled our van into that stall. Rather than go into the grocery store, I decided to remain outside in the sunlight. Pretty soon a man pulled his pickup truck into the crosshatched walkway. As he was walking to the store, I asked him not to park in the walkway. He ignored me and went into the store. When he came out of the store I went up to him as he was getting into his truck. He said that unless I was an officer of the law I had no right to criticize where he parked. I said that he was an absolute asshole. (I regretted this and I wish that I had said he was blocking access to my vehicle.) He called me "a fucking gimp." I thought of moving my wheelchair around to the back of his truck so that he couldn't pullout, but then I thought better of that as he might actually pull out.

Once, when we were in the cafeteria at the Grand Canyon, I was trying to order something from one of the food servers. Things were very busy and she was being stressed by people pressing her for orders while she was lacking food from the kitchen. Anyhow, she was repeatedly and completely ignoring me as though I didn't exist, though I was calling to her as loudly as I could.

I go for "walks" around the neighborhood. My wheelchair is controlled by sipping and puffing into a tube. Perhaps you may ask how I can both turn and control speed with just sipping and puffing. A hard puff starts the chair forward. It keeps going until I pull my mouth away from the tube. I can make a right turn by a soft blow, a left turn by a soft sip. A hard sip starts me going backward. Continued hard puffs or sips ramps up the speed.

I sometimes meet up with a cat named "Rocky." Rocky belongs to owners of the Weatherford Hotel. I call for Rocky and he comes and jumps onto my lap. I give him a ride for about 30 feet, which is all that he will tolerate.

Once, a milkweed thistle blew into my ear on one of my walks. Arrrgh! This goes along with an itch on the nose, a fly on the face, or a bee buzzing around. There is nothing that a quadriplegic can do except try to ignore them.

One time I was going along the right side of a street when up ahead a van was backing out of a driveway on the other side of the street. I stopped about 60 feet short of the driveway so as not to be in the driver's way. But the driver kept coming despite my yelling. The reason for this was a car that was ahead of him in the driveway and wanted to get out. The van passed me with about

1-foot clearance and went so far back that I was even with the driver's seat. I was still yelling. but I got no acknowledgement from the driver in the closed up van. Incidentally, I was only two feet from the edge of the road.

In 1995, we decided to follow up our trip on the Delta Queen with a trip on the American Queen. We went on its maiden voyage from Pittsburgh, Pennsylvania down the Allegheny to the Ohio River and then up the Mississippi to St. Louis, Missouri where we spent the fourth of July. Then we went down the Mississippi to New Orleans. Altogether, it was a 17-day trip and we had an awful lot of fun.

The boat was as large as it possibly could be in order to fit through the locks on the rivers and to fit under the bridges. Its smokestacks, (yes, it really was a steamboat) hinged in the middle and could be tilted downward so that they would fit under the bridges. The Ohio River was not navigable throughout the year until the locks and associated dams were built to hold back the water so that boats would not run aground. The locks are under the authority of the Army Corps of Engineers. You may remember the story in the newspapers about the American Queen running aground on a sandbar. The Delta Queen Steamboat Co., who owns the American Queen, claim that the Army Corps of Engineers let the water get too low in the river. Anyhow, it took several days to get the boat off of the sandbar.

The American Queen has several elevators that run between the five decks. Inasmuch as our cabin was on the highest deck that was accessible to the elevators and the dining room was two decks below, I depended on the elevators. Occasionally, the elevators would get stuck. The maintenance crew blamed the elevator problems on the fact that the boat had become stuck on the sand bar which warped the hull of the boat and distorted the alignment of the elevator shafts.

Of course, one of the main pleasures of being on a cruise is eating. They had marvelous food. On the last two days, they did repeat the dinner menu. However, sometimes we skipped dinner because we ate hot dogs in late afternoon at the stern of the boat where there was also a bar. The hot dogs were some of the best I have ever tasted. From the stern, we could watch the paddle wheel and the birds following in the wake of the boat. Breakfast was served in what they called "The Front Porch of America." This was an open deck at the bow of the boat. Part of it was enclosed, hence the name "Front Porch."

We had charming dinner companions. One couple was from California, another couple was from Florida, and the lady who sat across from me, who was in a wheelchair, would have three martinis straight up each dinnertime. She was up in her 80's and accompanied by her daughter. I would have my martini on the rocks, but one was enough for me.

This trip taught us a lot about traveling. It taught us to make sure all the arrangements were tied down. We flew to Pittsburgh where we were supposed to be picked up by a handicap van. They had an ordinary bus to carry all the passengers. It could not take a wheelchair because it did not have a lift. We had tried to specify a lift, but no, they thought they could get by with the bus. Handicap vans were not available because they had to be ordered 24 hours in advance. But there was no way that I could get to the hotel without one. After about 2 1/2 hours, they were able to get me a van.

The flight to Pittsburgh on United Airlines went very well. We had a monstrous array of baggage though. One of the items was a commode chair that was broken down so that the back was removed and stored inside. The thing looked like a box on wheels. Of course, the hole was plugged up and we had stuff stored inside. I pushed the commode with a big suitcase on wheels in front of it across the glazed floor and around the zigzag passenger check-in lines. Of course, I did the pushing with my powered wheelchair.

We made our return trip from New Orleans on Continental Airlines. This was almost a disaster. First of all, the plane from New Orleans to Dallas-Fort Worth was canceled and we had to take a plane to Houston that upset the remaining part of our reservations to Phoenix. We had a several hour delay and we had to move to another terminal for the connecting flight. It was at this point that I discovered that they had broken my wheelchair. The control wires from the joystick were broken, and there was damage to one of the wheels. The airline furnished us with an attendant to push the wheelchair over to the other terminal. All the while on the trip over there, the guy who was pushing me, told me that it was a shame that I let my muscles get into such poor shape. I didn't explain to him that it was impossible for me to exercise if my nerves didn't work. Anyhow, it was all very unpleasant.

In Houston, the safety officer decided to check whether the batteries in my wheelchair were certified for flying. I assured him that they were sealed gel cells and were certified for air worthiness. It took a lot of arguing to convince him that we could continue with our journey. After several hours of delay, we could make our connection to Phoenix. After being completely exhausted by all of this, we finally arrived in Phoenix. On the following, day we drove back to Flagstaff.

It was a number of years before we made another long trip. The occasion was the 50th reunion of my Johns Hopkins University class of 1949. We used the Internet to search for the best way that I might make the trip. We contacted several different travel agencies that specialized in arranging travel for handicapped people. One recommended that we go by air because all the discomfort would be over in several hours. But we recognized that this assumed that there would be no cancellation of flights or weather delays. One travel agency recommended that we go by train from Tucson to Jacksonville, Florida and then north on one of the Miami-New York express trains. But this would have entailed driving to Tucson, a distance of 280 miles. Anyhow, they made very clear to us that we should tie down every aspect of the trip. Marge made the Amtrak reservations, as well as hotel reservations, and an arrangement for handicapped van travel from Washington to Baltimore and also in Baltimore. Since Amtrak's Southwestern Chief goes through Flagstaff and thence to Chicago, we elected to take the handicap-accessible room on this train. From Chicago, after a several hour wait, we could get the Capital Limited to Washington D.C. We arranged for a train to Baltimore, a distance of only 40 miles, but then we didn't make that connection and opted instead to take the handicap van to Baltimore. This took us straight to our hotel.

Actually, the car from Chicago to Washington was exactly the same car that we took from Flagstaff and we had the same room assignment. Marge had nailed this down six months in advance. However, we had to get off in Chicago in order that they could clean the train and for this they had to move it out of the station. They let us keep stuff in our room which was very lucky because I don't know how we would have stored it all.

One item was the pink monster. This was a foam mattress that would substitute for a hospital bed that had its feet up and its head raised at about a 15 degree angle. At that time, my wheelchair was very long because the ventilator and a storage battery to power it were supported on a back porch to the chair. As a result, when I was in my room on the train, my feet stuck into the aisle. This was the largest room on the train. In order to get me into bed, I had to maneuver my chair down the narrow aisle to the vestibule where there was room to get me into the Hoyer. Marge would push me back to the room and Tina (who went along to help with all these activities) would move me over to the pink monster where I spent the night.

The porter would bring dinner from the dining room. For one dinner, I ordered the Southwestern Special, which was a Navajo taco (a deep fried leavened taco with black beans and sour cream on top). Well, somehow because of our crowding, Tina put my plate on the seat and then forgetting about it, she proceeded to sit on it. But we managed to survive this way.

We arrived in Washington in pretty good shape and were only about 1 1/2 hours late. The company that was to provide the van was aware of the situation and waited for our phone call to bring the van around. The rest of the trip to Baltimore was uneventful.

The Class of 1949 had decided that it would sponsor several lectures by Johns Hopkins professors. A week or two before leaving Flagstaff, I was asked by one of the Hopkins staff if I would introduce one of the speakers, Prof. Richard C. Henry, who is Professor of Astrophysics. This I agreed to do. It was fortunate that Dick Henry had a web site that had all sorts of interesting information about him. I memorized the spiel that I would make because it would have been awkward to hold up written notes. I requested a microphone, which was provided, and also made sure that there were no impediments to my getting to the microphone. The introduction went pretty well. I forgot to say a few things that I meant to, but that's always the case with me. After the lectures, I had lunch with Professor Henry. Actually, we had never met before, but then he is into the expanding universe and I am into planets.

Being back in my home town was very enjoyable. We went to Haussner's Restaurant, which was famous nationally for good German food and for its extensive art collection, which covered every available bit of wall space. I ordered hassenpheffir, a dish they were famous for. Unfortunately, the restaurant had lost a lot of business to restaurants at Harbor Place, the new waterfront mall. Haussner's was forced to close last year.

We stayed at The Colonnade, which is very close to the University. We could walk to most of the buildings where the various class meetings were. Marge had arranged for a hospital bed to be placed in our room, so we didn't have to deal with the pink monster.

The 1949 Class Reunion banquet was a dinner cruise from Harbor Place down the Patapsico River. Marge had ascertained that the boat would be accessible to my wheelchair. When we got there, we found that there was a 6-inch high scupper around the deck. They summoned four goons to lift my chair over the scupper. Well, before I could stop them, they were grabbing the leg supports and the armrests. They ended up bending the leg supports. Generally, people don't realize that these parts of a wheelchair are fragile and the chair should be lifted by its frame.

The dinner was very enjoyable. I had crab, also a favorite. I met some of my old classmates, Tom Frost, Per Gloersen, and others. We spent a long time going over old stories and more recent events. As far as the cruise went, it was very good and we went down as far as the Chesapeake Bay Bridge.

All of the Reunion Classes had their banquet dinner together at the Baltimore Museum of Art, which is on the edge of the Hopkins campus. It was a fairly good dinner that was catered. I was surprised when people began coming up to me and thanked me for the "marvelous" introduction that I made for Professor Henry. One person even said it was world class. I've never been thanked for an introduction before. I was amazed. It gave me a very good feeling about the effort that I, and particularly Marge, had made in making such a long trip for me.

We ate a couple of dinners at the restaurant at the Colonnade. The first time we ate there, everything went very well. However, the second time I had somewhat of a distasteful encounter when being seated. The hostess directed us to a table that was perfectly satisfactory, but as I was pulling up to the table the manager, a short stout buxom woman in a bright red dress, came up and directed us to a table farther back from the door. I protested that the table that we were at was perfectly fine. But the woman said "Sir, I'm doing this so that you will be more comfortable." She began seating us, but then decided another table, still farther back, was better. I again protested that the second table was fine, but again the woman said "Sir, I'm doing this so that you will be more comfortable." Now, we were behind a large column and couldn't be seen from the front door. I would have walked out but there were no other restaurants in the vicinity. The food was very good. Marge had filet mignon. I had a bite of this and I think it is one of the best filets I've ever tasted. I had a dinner of shad and shad roe. I hadn't had shad roe for years. My mother used to fix it if it was in season when I came to Baltimore. I think it's marvelous but it is very rich. Well, I enjoyed that dinner despite the altercation with the manager.

Finally, it was time to go back to Flagstaff. We again got a van to take us to Washington. The driver picked us up early so that we would have time to make a short tour of Washington, D.C. We also had time to have lunch in Union Station. We ate in a food court. There was a seafood stand that had raw oysters on the half shell. I ordered a half dozen of the oysters, which Tina fed to me. She wondered if I swallowed them whole. I told her that no, I chewed them up because I enjoyed the taste and texture. It is impossible to describe the taste, but the texture varies from chewy for the frilly muscle part to mealy for the body part. They really were very good oysters. I hadn't had any like those for 30 years.

We were supposed to arrive back in Flagstaff at about 9:00 p.m. three nights later but didn't arrive until after 1:00 a.m. Believe it or not, we arrived in a snowstorm and this was in late April. It has been known to snow in Flagstaff in June. We had arranged to be picked up in my Dodge Caravan and our driver still met us at the station despite the late hour.

I don't think that I should try flying. Some of the delays that have been reported for airline travel would have completely depleted all the battery power that I have available for my ventilator. It is too scary to travel with such a possible disaster. Either I travel by train, or travel by my van, but I don't think I should try traveling by commercial airline.

Research, Cures and
Palliative Care for ALS

Recent research on ALS has made some startling breakthroughs in understanding some aspects of the disease. There seems, however, to be many causes for ALS, and, in any event, it is a very complicated disease. Here, for the most part, I will follow some exciting threads of current research. A lot of my discussion on this is based upon a document received from Will Klausmeier by e-mail. Dr. Klausmeier is not a physician but is a medical chemist and he provides a disclaimer, as do I, for responsibility for any proposed treatment given here. I do not have the background to provide any recommendations on courses of treatment.

I have been trying to keep up with some of the research being done on ALS and I can document some of the discussion given by Klausmeier. The research abstracts that I have seen are full of jargon and consequently are difficult to follow. Klausmeier gives a glossary of terms that is, to say the least, enlightening.

I will first give a short review of what was known about ALS up until 1995. Some of this may overlap that which was given in a previous chapter, but I think that some repetition is needed here because of the complexity of the subject. It has been known that in the upper and lower motor neurons the message is carried across the gap, called the synapse, between successive neurons by glutamate. After transporting the message, the glutamate is absorbed by glial cells that convert the glutamate to glutamine and transport it back to the presynaptic neuron where it is converted back to glutamate and stored in vesicles of the presynaptic neuron. In the case of persons with ALS, the glutamate is not entirely disposed of. The build up of glutamate continues to excite the succeeding neuron which eventually dies because of repeating excitation. This effect is called excitotoxicity.

I believe that a breakthrough discovery was made in 1995 by Dr. Jeffrey Rothstein of the Johns Hopkins University Medical School. He discovered a protein, which he called EAAT2 and which stands for excitotoxic amino acid transporter number 2. Since either way this is quite a mouthful, I am going to refer to this as the glutamate bus. This protein is manufactured by messenger RNA which is produced from the DNA of a specific gene. He found that the gene was not defective in sporadic ALS patients, but for some reason the messenger RNA produced an incorrect protein. He found that the glutamate bus protein is 30-95% reduced in patients with sporadic ALS. The glutamate bus is contained in the wall of the glial cell. Its role is to transport the glutamate to the inside of the cell. With reduced amount of the glutamate bus in PALS, the glutamate builds up in the synapses. It was also found that in the case of the patients with the SOD1 defect, free radicals produced by the enzyme damaged the glutamate bus so that it was ineffective in transporting the glutamate.

A recent discovery was made by Dr. Martina M. Berger of the University of California at Irvine. She found that tissue from the spinal cords of sporadic ALS patients contained an enterovirus. This virus, called echo-7, was found in 88% of the ALS patients. As convincing as this may sound, other researchers have found evidence of different viruses. After all, the presence of a virus does not mean that it is the cause of the disease. There is some evidence for a herpes-like virus and other indications are of slow acting viruses similar to the polio virus. At the present time, some clinics are prescribing a "cocktail" of a mixture of anti-viral drugs that include pleconaril, effective against enteroviruses, and ganclovir or acyclovir, which are effective against retroviruses such as the herpes virus. But just finding viruses in the spinal cords of PALS is no proof that it is the causative agent.

There are many avenues of research that are presently being pursued. I believe that the above scheme leaves many questions unanswered. For example, is glutamate toxicity the only cause of motor neuron death? What, precisely, is the mechanism for neuronal death? Are environmental factors important? It seems to me that pesticides, herbicides, solvents, mercury and lead exposures may cause some cases. About 10% of ALS cases are familial. But apparently, only 20% of these cases are caused by the defective SOD1 gene. What are the causes of the other 80% of familial cases? A very recent discovery suggests that another gene is responsible for some of the ALS cases where dementia is involved.

If the causal factors are removed from a patient, then the neurons will need to be replaced even though neurons regenerate at a very slow rate. Hopefully, the way has now been cleared for human stem cell research to be conducted in the U.S. It is hoped that transplantation of stem cells will regenerate new neurons. Recent work has shown recovery of function in ALS mice. But much research needs to be done before stem cells can be used for human patients. Where and how should they be introduced? What precautions should be taken? How should their effectiveness be monitored? The future does look bright for cures and effective treatment of ALS cases. Continued funding of research at an enhanced level is certain to produce results.

Care for persons with ALS and spinal cord injuries has continued to improve. It used to be that these people were sent home to die. I still experience this concept in my care. For example, a physical therapist said to me that she didn't recommend a powered wheelchair for ALS patients; I presume because she assumed we didn't live long enough. Consider Medicare's policy on ventilators. They only rent them. I presume they considered that it was not economical to purchase one. They have rented mine for nearly four years. It has been more than paid for.

Some doctors that are involved with the care of ALS patients have stated that with proper care ALS patients need not die from pneumonia or respiratory infection. The end of their life will be determined by the usual causes such as cardiac disease, stroke, or cancer. ALS patients eventually need some kind of mechanical ventilation and with this, there is a need for 24-hour caregiving. This is expensive and is not covered by Medicare. Caregivers do not need to be registered nurses or respiratory therapists. The patient placed on ventilation is provided with training for their primary caregiver when they leave the hospital. I suggest that CNAs or others be hired for their training in transferring patients and range of motion exercising and then these people be trained by the primary caregiver in the procedures of suctioning the trachea and the operation in connection to the ventilator. Of course, regular visits to a pulmonologist are required. All this care is expensive and it is also a nuisance. It is a matter of choice for each patient whether the quality of life is sufficient to justify the expense. But I have certainly found that my life continues to be rewarding.

The conclusion that many PALS need not die from respiratory failure is so astonishing that I feel that I should support it with references to professional papers even though this is not customary in a popular level book. (See Appendix C for these references.) I believe that I can't overstress the fact that many can choose to live. I've read that an ALS nursing consultant has said that there is no reason for persons with ALS to die if they are given adequate care. I don't believe that this view is shared by many pulmonologists. Many ALS patients could live longer than they have in the past.

Recently, a new ventilator became available for home use. It is made by Pulmonetics, and, in my opinion, it is a great improvement over the Respironics respirator that Medicare rented for me. It is much smaller, about the size of a laptop computer. It is based on a new technology that doesn't use a large piston or bellows that are normally used to displace its volume of air into the lungs. Instead, it uses a high speed turbine to quickly push the air into the lungs for each breath. The company that makes this is a small startup company which cannot afford to loan out machines on a rental basis. We could not find a company to take on the loan, so we had to purchase it. It cost more than $13,000, but it has been worth it. My wheelchair no longer has to have the back porch to support the large Respironics ventilator. This back porch stuck out about 18 inches and was always getting in the way when I was making turns or backing up. It didn't allow for me to get into in my Caravan properly. Now, with my new ventilator, I can get into the van easily. It is no problem for me to go down to coffee.

I recently got home health (Medicare) to come help me with the exercises for my neck. Their requirement was that I not go out except for a doctor's appointment. What negative thinking that is! The requirement is that I be home-bound. Hopefully, they will change the definition of home-bound to include those that require the assistance of others to go out.

The situation is improving. For example, the new ventilator was invented precisely for the purpose of allowing more freedom for people to get outside. Their advertising literature shows a girl on horseback with a ventilator slung over her shoulder like a handbag. I hope it won't be long before Medicare will be able to rent, or better yet, purchase these ventilators.

Persons with tracheostomies need to be very careful about avoiding respiratory tract infections. An infection can lead to pneumonia which may be fatal. One thing that helps me to avoid infections is that all the air that I breathe is filtered through a micro filter. The infections that I have had were readily cured by antibiotics. I hope that I don't run into an intractable bronchial infection.

Computers have given great capability to many PALS. Stephen Hawking has been able to carry on his research in theoretical astrophysics and even to give lectures using a computer produced voice. He has been on Larry King Live show and in movies and TV shows. I sometimes encounter this computer-generated voice at conventions displaying assistive devices and I can't help but think that Stephen Hawking must be there.

New mattress design and newer cushions for wheelchairs make it possible to avoid pressure sores called decubitus. I have been in a wheelchair for nearly six years and I have not yet suffered a pressure sore except for a tiny one on a toe. They are avoidable.

With these improvements in care, PALS are living longer and happier. And even before cures, people with ALS have an outlook for improved quality of life.

Some of My Car Treks

Since I can't travel by air, then I must travel by car to those places where Amtrak doesn't go. It is difficult for Marge and me to travel more than 250 to 300 miles per day. It takes us an hour and a half to get up and get breakfast in the morning. It takes equally long or longer at night. Of course, Marge has to do all of this for me so this does not include her time. So car travel is slow but there are few uncertainties.

The most important device that enabled us to make extended car trips is the Pulmonetics ventilator. Its small size allows my wheelchair to fit properly into the Dodge Caravan. We are also able to store the cart on which we carry the Respironics ventilator (I don't dare go without a backup), suction machine, and all the other stuff that I need. The Hoyer lift fits into the van too. It straddles the cart. The backseat of the car was filled up with suitcases and the pink monster.

Our first long trip after becoming ventilator dependent was the trip Marge and I had planned when I wound up in the emergency room before my tracheotomy nearly four years earlier. This was a trip to Death Valley and the California Railroad Museum in Sacramento. At the end of the trip, we swung down to Pasadena where I attended the annual meeting of the Division of Planetary Sciences of the American Astronomical Society.

I know that I mentioned this earlier but it continues to come back to us that all arrangements should be tied down before beginning a trip. This is even of greater necessity with car travel because more nights and more different lodgings are involved. Here are some of the problems we have encountered that we didn't anticipate.

On our way back from Pasadena, we spent a night in Needles, California, and we didn't make a motel reservation because there are so many motels there. It turned out that we had a difficult time finding a motel that didn't have platform beds (beds with boards along the sides and ends so that the maids do not have to clean underneath). Our problem with platform beds is that the wheels of the Hoyer will not fit underneath. Marge has been able to tilt the Hoyer so I swing over the bed, but this is a decidedly dangerous operation. With the help of one motel clerk in Needles, who took our plight to heart and phoned around to other motels, we found a place to stay.

On another trip, we found out that some reservation clerks will lie or at least not tell you the whole truth over the phone in order to get your business. We were promised that the bed would allow the Hoyer to go underneath. It was a platform bed. Moreover, the handicapped-accessible room had a 6-inch high step at the doorway. The room had support bars at the toilet and shower, but that is all that qualified it for being handicapped-accessible. I understand that the American Disability Act left it up to individual states to define the requirements for accessibility. Also, we found that the person making the reservations may not be in the same city as the motel.

One simple thing that seems to be overlooked in just about all handicapped rooms is the hindrance that is caused by automatic door closers. Typically, there is a narrow hallway from the doorway past the bathroom and closet to the bedroom. The door opens inward. If you are trying to go out, you are fighting the door closer as you try to hold the door while backing up in the wheelchair. Since Marge opens the door for me, there is nowhere for her to go to get out of my way. The solution is for us to take along a door wedge if we can remember this. Failing this, Marge uses her handbag to block the door open.

One of the big attractions for me on such a trip is the food. All sorts of food is available depending on locale. Fish is, of course, best near the coast so I was looking forward to this on our California trip. I was looking forward to lunch aboard the Delta King in Sacramento.

The Delta King was originally the "sister" boat of the Delta Queen. They both began service in 1927 in overnight passenger service between Sacramento and San Francisco. They both were commissioned in 1941 as training ships for the U. S. Navy and then as troop carriers down to ocean ports in the bay area.

In 1946, the Delta Queen was sold to the Thomas Greene Company of New Orleans. Its superstructure was boarded up and it was towed through the Panama Canal to New Orleans,where it was restored. Eventually it became the flagship of The Delta Queen Steamboat Company. The Congressional Safety at Sea Act of 1966, which required that vessels used in overnight passenger traffic have steel superstructures, nearly ended its career. Only last minute lobbying provided that an exemption be made for the Delta Queen. No such exemption was made for the Delta King, however. So the Delta King, which is operated by the Delta King Hotel Co., is restricted to being operated as a hotel and restaurant while remaining tied at a dock in Old Sacramento. So having lunch on the Delta King was a must. Of course, I had fish, and this time, catfish from the Sacramento river.

The major reason for going to Sacramento was so that I could visit The California Railroad Museum. There are some unique steam locomotives there. One is the C. P. Huntington, the first engine on the Central Pacific Railroad. It is unusual in having only two driving wheels. This turned out to be very impractical because of the lack of traction.

Another engine of historical significance is one of the cab-forward Southern Pacific oil burning locomotives. This railroad has numerous snow sheds and tunnels in the Sierra Nevada mountains. With a conventionally arranged locomotive having the smokestack in the front, the smoke would become overwhelming in the cab. Their solution was to turn the engine around with the cab, now enclosed with windows, up front. Since these were oil-burning locomotives, the oil could be pumped from the trailing tender to the firebox, which was also in front.

The next day we went on to Pasadena for the Division of Planetary Sciences meeting. We stayed at the Holiday Inn. For dinner the first evening, I ordered seared tuna. This seems to be a dish that is becoming very popular. The tuna is flash cooked to a depth of about 1/8-inch so that the interior remains raw. The fish must be of sashimi grade, otherwise there may be parasites in the meat. The Japanese call raw fish sashimi, not sushi as many Americans seem to think. Sushi is rice rolled in seaweed and may contain many different items other than fish rolled in its interior such as squid, octopus, crab or avocado (California sushi) to name a few.

Marge and I became quite familiar with sashimi when we were in Hawaii. Marge had a co-worker who moonlighted as a fish broker. Sometimes she had an excess of ahi (Hawaiian name for tuna). Marge would bring home about a pound of it and we would pig out. We ate it atop crackers with a little wasabi. Wasabi is a very strong Japanese horseradish. A bit about the size of a pea will nearly blow the top of your head off.

At the DPS convention, I took in some of the sessions, but particularly the one devoted to Io. I also took in a session of presentation of poster papers. This gave me more opportunities to meet many old friends. But the highlight of the meeting for me was the banquet and the preceding cocktail hour where I could talk at length to special friends. Altogether, I visited with more than 30 friends at the meeting. At the banquet dinner, I had salmon. Not only is this a very tasty fish, but it is rich in omega 3 fatty acids, which are good for you.

In May of 2001, we made a trip to Austin, Texas for the wedding of our youngest son, Alan. This trip took us four days each way with places to visit along the way. One of our first stops was at the Very Large Array radio telescope, which is near Soccoro, New Mexico. I had never visited this telescope before. One attraction was that it was the locale for much of the action in the movie "Contact".

San Antonio is the name of a very small town near to Soccoro. We made a point to stop at the Owl Bar and Cafe in the middle of the town. Their green chili cheeseburgers are marvelous. In 1945, the director of the Los Alamos National Laboratory, J. Robert Oppenheimer, who was working on preparations for the first test of an atom bomb at the nearby Trinity test site, convinced the owners of a small grocery store in San Antonio that he and his coworkers needed a place to eat. Thus, the Owl Bar and Cafe began. We made a point to stop there again on the way back for more green chili cheeseburgers.

Most states have state birds, trees, flowers and the like, but New Mexico has a state question, "Red or green?" I was asked this in a restaurant when ordering an enchilada. The question refers to whether I wanted red or green chili sauce.

The wedding came off marvelously. A special thrill for me was seeing my four year old grandson, Aaron, in a tuxedo. He was the ringbearer. He marched down the aisle with aplomb. The decision Marge and I made four years earlier to have the tracheotomy was surely the right one. Otherwise, I would never have witnessed Aaron in a tuxedo.

Whither Go-eth Bill

God

I have not used His name until now in this book. I am an atheist, but I am a member of a Unitarian Universalist Church. I suppose you might call me a humanist. I believe in the worth of every human being, all 6 billion. Also, I do not believe in a life after death. I believe that this life is it, and we had better do the best we can with it. We each have an obligation to make a contribution to humanity. Humanity has improved itself over its thousands of years of existence. I hope that this book will be part of my contribution. However, at this point in my life, I am not afraid to die.

When I was first diagnosed as having this terrible disease, I thought I would have only a couple years to live, but now I think I might live for a long time. My philosophy has always been to do the best that I can do rather than compete with other people. This way I can always be a winner. I need to pursue various projects to keep myself busy.

After I realized I couldn't do my large-scale model railroading any longer, I got back into ham radio. When the muscles in my hand got weaker and I could no longer send Morse code I prevailed upon Marge to build me a device that was described in the magazine *World Radio*. This device enables me to send Morse code simply by saying "dit daw," which the radio amateur uses instead of saying "dot dash." With this device, I can send about 18 words per minute. I use voice transmission as well. At the start of the year 2000, I worked toward getting the

Millennium Award from the American Radio Relay League. For this award, one needed to contact 100 countries in the year 2000. I contacted more than 100 countries in the first three months of 2000 which was great fun. About half my contacts were via Morse code. I have put off being on ham radio while writing this book. But since this is the last chapter, I will be getting back to ham radio pretty quickly. I am eager to get back on since sunspots are near their maximum in the 11-year-long solar cycle and this is the time for best transmission of radio signals worldwide.

Marge and I continue to go places by car. One recent trip was down to Phoenix to see a couple of Diamondbacks baseball games. PALS in Arizona can get invited to watch a game from Curt Shilling's (star pitcher) suite at Bank One Ballpark. Curt, and his wife Shonda, have done much to support research on ALS. I recently made a trip to Tucson to see Dr. Stern about whether some of the newer drugs might be useful for me to take. I came away with a renewed spirit. However, we ran into the same old problem of platform beds, despite being told that their handicapped room did not have them.

Aaron has developed into a bright young boy. I am so happy that I have lived long enough to really get to know him, and for him to know me. What a joy!

Lastly, it has been my purpose in writing this book to give courage to all the caregivers and to the sufferers of severe handicaps. I hope that I have helped some people.

"I've learned:

That life is like a roll of toilet paper. The closer it gets to the end, the faster it goes".

Andy Rooney

Epilogue
Marge's Story

I am Bill's wife and primary caregiver. My intention is to give a brief picture of what it has been like to be in both of these roles over the past eight years. It has been difficult, and because of this I have experienced significant personal growth.

After the diagnosis, I panicked. I was not ready to lose my husband. We talked and we cried. We made an agreement to go for broke - to spend money on equipment - to do everything we could to make our remaining time together as full as possible. It seemed to be a natural virtuous thing to give up many of my activities. Those activities were those things that gave me personal satisfaction. What could be more satisfying than taking care of the man I loved?

We did pretty well for a while.

Then, five months after Bill went on the ventilator, I was diagnosed with breast cancer and had my second mastectomy. Afterwards, I was depressed. I thought that I would be the first to die with nothing more in my life but caregiving. I did everything from brushing his hair to flossing his teeth to wiping his ass, but did very little for myself. I was not suicidal, but I was clear that I was unwilling to live my life as I had been.

Although I knew that none existed, I hoped my doctor could give me a magic pill that would make me do my caregiving duties with energy and enthusiasm. Well, there is no such pill. What she did insist on was that I get help on board at least five days a week and see a counselor. I took her advice and it helped; it kept me going. Bill felt me withdrawing from him emotionally. I had a lot of work to do.

We hired three wonderful people to help take care of Bill so that I could get out to take care of myself. However, as helpful as that was, having others in the house was an assault on my sense of privacy.

Through counseling, I was able to begin to deal with my feelings of resentment and frustration by paying more attention to how I felt about the things that we could not do because of ALS. I had to grieve these losses before I could focus on the things that we can do.

Bill cannot fly but an aide and I did get him on Amtrak for a cross country trip so that he could attend his 50th college reunion. It was a real adventure and we were so glad we did it. We also took a two week automobile trip to California. I was so tired and depressed that scenery went unnoticed and I became terrified of the California freeways. We drove to Austin, Texas to attend our youngest son's wedding. Our oldest son, Bob, helped with the driving and loading and unloading all of the stuff that you need when travelling with Bill. It was four days each way. The joy of the trip was that I felt that Bob knew what I was going through, really knew. We are closer now than we ever have been.

As I grieved my losses, my feelings of love and caring resurfaced. Bill is happier. I am happier. In fact, our communication is the best it has ever been.

At a recent Hospice sponsored teleconference on caregiving, I learned that fatigue is not only physical, but also mental and spiritual. I had forgotten about the spiritual side of my life.

My next task is to renew my spiritual energy.

After forty years of marriage and eight years of caregiving, 1 love my husband and feel privileged to be able to take care of him.

I Choose To Live

144

Appendix A

William M. Sinton

Antecedents traced back to 1640 in Armagh county in Ireland.

Great great grandfather James, emigrated to Richmond, VA. He was a candle and soap maker.

Great grandfather George F., was a comptroller on the B & O Railroad.

Grandfather Robert D., was a grain and feed broker.

Father Robert N. was a salesman of leather belting for machinery.

Birth date and Place: - 4/11/25, Baltimore, Maryland

Education:

Baltimore City Schools
AB, 1949, Johns Hopkins University
PhD, 1953, Johns Hopkins University

Married to Marjorie A. Korner, 1960, 3 children

Appointments:

Research Associate, Johns Hopkins
University, 1953-1954
Research Associate and Lecturer,
Harvard College Observatory, 1954-1957
Astrophysicist, Smithsonian Astrophysical Observatory, 1956-1957
Astronomer, Lowell Observatory, 1957-1966

Professor of Physics and Astronomy, Institute for
Astronomy, University of Hawaii, 1966-
1990, Retired
Adjunct Astronomer, Lowell Observatory, 1989-

Professional Societies:
Optical Society of America (Fellow)
American Astronomical Society, (Division of
Planetary Sciences - Committeeman, 1971-
1974)
International Astronomical Union
(Commission 16, Physical Study of Planets
and Satellites)

Awards and Honorary Societies:
Purple Heart Medal - 1944
Adolph Lomb Medal of the Optical Society
of America - 1954
Sigma Xi
Phi Beta Kappa

Listings:
Who's Who in America
Who's Who in the West
American Men and Women of Science
Men and Women of Hawaii
2000 Outstanding Scientists of 20th Century Inter-
national Biographical Society

Publications:

      More than 100 - topics: infrared instrumentation, planets and other astronomical studies and articles in popular magazines

      "Tools of the Astronomer," with G. R. Miczaika, Harvard University Press, Cambridge, MA, 1961.

Administrative Posts and Committees:

      Scientist in charge of Mauna Kea Observatory 1967-1971 (founding years). Established most of the policies that are still in effect.

      Co-Organizer of International Jupiter Watch (1986 - 1990), Discipline Leader of Satellite Discipline (1986-90).

      Member of Time Allocation Committee, NASA Infrared Telescope Facility (1991- 1993).

      Advisory Board for Lowell Observatory (1991-). Honorary Member (2000 -).

I Choose To Live

Appendix B

Mauna Kea Trail
Tune: Chisholm Trail, Words: W. M. Sinton, 1969

Come along boys, listen to my tale,
I'll tell you about my troubles on the Mauna Kea trail.

Come a ki-yi yippee yea yippee yea,
Come a ki-yi yippee yea.

A bumpy road and the dust in your eye,
Twenty-eight percent and a four-wheel drive.

Refrain

Your head is aching 'cause the air is thin,
Your only relief is the ox-y-gin.

Refrain

There's the top at fourteen thousand feet,
The clouds beneath you and ain't it neat

Refrain

Sirius and Canopus are high in the sky,
See the stars for more then two pi[1].

Refrain

Your head is aching cause the air is thin,
You're only relief is the as-pir-in.

Refrain

The sky is clear and the water vapor is low,
Measure many stars not seen by Frank Low[2].

Refrain

[1] A hemisphere is a solid angle of 2π. Hence, more than two pi implies being able to see downward to the horizon.

[2] Frank Low was then an astronomer at the University of Arizona and specialized in infrared studies.

Appendix C

References, Web Sites and E-mail Addresses

1. Bach, J.R.: Amyotrophic lateral sclerosis. Communication status and survival with ventilatory support. Am J Phys Med Rehabil, (1993). 72(6): p. 343-9. Abstract: The use of ventilatory support via an indwelling tracheotomy tube in the management of advanced amyotrophic lateral sclerosis patients demands the commitment of enormous resources. The use of non-invasive respiratory aids can facilitate and simplify home management, decrease expense and prepare patients and families for decision making regarding tracheotomy if and when this becomes necessary. The purposes of this study were to: describe the utility of non-invasive respiratory aids, determine to what extent survival might be expected to increase by the use of mechanical ventilation, and explore the consequences of patient disposition and communication status on survival. Eighty-nine patients survived a mean of 4.4 +/- 3.9 yr (range = 1 month to 26.5 yr) using respiratory support. This included 37 patients who were still alive. The "up to 24 h use of non-invasive intermittent positive pressure ventilation" (IPPV) methods delayed or eliminated tracheotomy for 25 patients. Survival was comparable for patients maintained at home or in chronic care facilities. The maintenance of effective communication appeared to favor patients remaining in the community. It could not be shown to affect survival, but it greatly increased quality of

life. The use of non-invasive respiratory muscle aids can eliminate the need for crisis decision-making regarding tracheotomy for many individuals with ALS.

2. Norris, F.H.: Care of the amyotrophic lateral sclerosis patient, in Amyotrophic lateral sclerosis: A comprehensive guide to management, Hiroshi Mitsumoto and Forbes H. Norris, Jr., Editors. 1994, Demos: New York. p. 29-42.

3. Norris, F.H. and R.J. Fallat: Respiratory Function, in Motor Neuron Disease, A.C. Williams, Editor. 1994, Chapman & Hall Medical: New York. p. 239-264.

4. Oppenheimer, E.A.: Decision-making in the respiratory care of amyotrophic lateral sclerosis: should home mechanical ventilation be used? Palliat Med, (1993). 7 (4 Suppl): p. 49-64. Abstract: As respiratory function starts to deteriorate in those with amyotrophic lateral sclerosis, one of the principal questions that has to be answered is whether it it is appropriate to provide ventilatory support. Although expensive, it is perfectly feasible to provide this at home, and this article examines many of the issues surrounding home mechanical ventilation.

5. Oppenheimer, E.A.: Respiratory management and home mechanical ventilation in amyotrophic lateral sclerosis., in Amyotrophic lateral sclerosis: A comprehensive guide to management, H.a.N. Mitsumoto F.H., Editor. 1994, Demos: New York. p. 139-165.

6. Edward Anthony Oppenheimer: Amyotrophic Lateral Sclerosis: Care, survival and quality of life on home mechanical ventilation. Chapter in book: Home Mechanical Ventilation (T.N. Willig, Editor). Arnette-Blackwell Publishers (1995); pages 249-260.

7. Pamela A. Cazzolli and Edward A. Oppenheimer: Home mechanical ventilation for Amyotrophic Lateral Sclerosis (ALS): Nasal compared to tracheotomy intermittent positive pressure ventilation (IPPV). (J. Neurol. Sci. - pending publication).

8. Hayashi, H., S. Kato, and A. Kawada: Amyotrophic lateral sclerosis patients living beyond respiratory failure. J Neurol Sci, (1991). 105(1): p. 73-8. Abstract: Thirty cases of amyotrophic lateral sclerosis (ALS) supported by respirators for more than 1 year beyond respiratory failure were followed to estimate the progression of their voluntary motor impairment. The extremities were apt to be affected within two years of the onset of the disease, but complete voluntary paralysis occurred in less than half of the cases (14/30), more frequently appearing after respiratory failure. Respiratory and bulbar paralysis were closely related, and combined complete voluntary paralysis of these muscle systems was observed in 25/30 cases. Incomplete external ophthalmoplegia also increased after respiratory failure, but complete voluntary external ophthalmoplegia was rare (5/30).

The ALS Association – USA – National Office
27001 Agoura Road, Suite 150
Calabasas Hills, CA 91301-5104
TEL (818) 880-9007

E-Mail: alsinfo@alsa-national.org
www.alsa.org

Bob Broedel's ALS Digest:
>To subscribe, to unsubscribe, to contribute notes,
>etc. to ALS Digest, please send e-mail to:
>bro@huey.met.fsu.edu

Appendix C